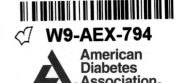
Teens with Diabetes:
A Clinician's Guide

Developmental Demands • Self-Management • Relationships • Transition

Michael A. Harris, PhD; Korey K. Hood, PhD; and Jill Weissberg-Benchell, PhD, CDE

Director, Book Publishing, Abe Ogden; *Managing Editor,* Greg Guthrie; *Acquisitions Editor,* Victor Van Beuren; *Project Manager,* Wendy M. Martin-Shuma; *Production Manager,* Melissa Sprott; *Composition,* ADA; *Cover Design,* Kim Woody; *Printer,* Data Reproductions.

Printed in the United States of America

1 3 5 7 9 10 8 6 4 2

The suggestions and information contained in this publication are generally consistent with the *Clinical Practice Recommendations* and other policies of the American Diabetes Association, but they do not represent the policy or position of the Association or any of its boards or committees. Reasonable steps have been taken to ensure the accuracy of the information presented. However, the American Diabetes Association cannot ensure the safety or efficacy of any product or service described in this publication. Individuals are advised to consult a physician or other appropriate health care professional before undertaking any diet or exercise program or taking any medication referred to in this publication. Professionals must use and apply their own professional judgment, experience, and training and should not rely solely on the information contained in this publication before prescribing any diet, exercise, or medication. The American Diabetes Association—its officers, directors, employees, volunteers, and members—assumes no responsibility or liability for personal or other injury, loss, or damage that may result from the suggestions or information in this publication.

⊗ The paper in this publication meets the requirements of the ANSI Standard Z39.48-1992 (permanence of paper).

ADA titles may be purchased for business or promotional use or for special sales. To purchase more than 50 copies of this book at a discount, or for custom editions of this book with your logo, contact the American Diabetes Association at the address below, at booksales@diabetes. org, or by calling 703-299-2046.

American Diabetes Association
1701 North Beauregard Street
Alexandria, Virginia 22311

DOI: 10.2337/9781580405317

Library of Congress Cataloging-in-Publication Data
Harris, Michael A. (Michael Avram), author.
 Teens with diabetes : a clinician's guide / Michael A. Harris, Korey K. Hood, Jill Weissberg-Benchell.
  p. ; cm.
 Includes bibliographical references and index.
 ISBN 978-1-58040-531-7 (alk. paper)
 I. Hood, Korey K., author. II. Weissberg-Benchell, Jill, author. III. American Diabetes Association, issuing body. IV. Title.
 [DNLM: 1. Diabetes Mellitus--psychology. 2. Adolescent Development. 3. Adolescent. 4. Parent-Child Relations. 5. Self Care. WK 810]
 RJ420.D5
 616.4'6200835--dc23
          2013042491

Contents

Foreword

Diabetes is the second most prevalent chronic disease in childhood, occurring in about one of every 400–500 people below the age of 20 years in the United States. The prevalence of diabetes in this age-group is second only to that of asthma. Diabetes is a lifelong disease, and children with diabetes become adolescents with diabetes and then adults with diabetes. In adults, diabetes is a leading cause of new-onset blindness (due to diabetic retinopathy), renal failure (resulting in the need for dialysis or renal transplantation), nontraumatic amputations, and macrovascular disease (contributing to cerebrovascular [stroke] or coronary artery [heart attack] disease). According to the Centers for Disease Control and Prevention, in 2012, diabetes was the seventh leading cause of death in the U.S. and was a major contributor to the first (heart disease), fourth (cerebrovascular disease), and eighth (renal disease) leading causes. Therefore, overall, diabetes is a devastating disorder.

Metabolic control of diabetes (mostly, but not exclusively, glycemic/glucose control) is clearly associated with the long-term outcomes of diabetes. Better glycemic control, as determined by hemoglobin A1C, when started relatively early in the course of diabetes (even during adolescence), reduces the subsequent risks of retinopathy, nephropathy, neuropathy, and macrovascular disease. Although this fact has been clearly demonstrated for type 1 diabetes by the Diabetes Control and Complications Trial (DCCT)/Epidemiology of Diabetes

Interventions and Complications (EDIC) Study and for type 2 diabetes by the U.K. Diabetes Prospective Study (UKPDS), morbidity and mortality associated with long-term diabetes complications still occur at an unacceptable rate.

Despite advancing knowledge over recent decades, the physiology of glucose metabolism and the pathophysiology of diabetes are not completely understood. Even after more than 90 years since the discovery and initial use of insulin to treat diabetes by Banting and Best, normalization of metabolic control remains an elusive goal for most people with type 1 and many with type 2 diabetes. For type 1 diabetes, which most commonly starts during childhood and depends on insulin replacement as the mainstay of treatment, the development of improved insulins and insulin analogs, self-monitoring of blood glucose (SMBG), and continuous glucose monitoring (CGM) and insulin pumps (continuous subcutaneous insulin infusion [CSII]) has significantly improved long-term outcomes and quality of life. However, normalization of metabolic control is still not a reality for most.

Managing diabetes requires attention to detail to a complex and changing medical regimen, usually multiple times a day. Diabetes management affects and is affected by every aspect of daily life. There is no vacation from the procedures related to diabetes management. Perhaps more than any other chronic disease of childhood, with the possible exception of asthma, diabetes requires continuous attention by the individual and his or her family and caregivers. The complex nature and imperfection of insulin replacement and the diabetes management regimen place substantial burdens on patients and their families. This burden is present at all ages and stages of life with different implications at each stage. However, these burdens are most challenging during adolescence. The nature of adolescence and the struggles prominent during this stage of psychosocial development conflict with the demands and continual immersion required to optimize metabolic control of diabetes. And even when implemented diligently, the results may be less than anticipated. *Clearly, there is more to optimal diabetes management than providing the right amount of insulin at the correct times relative to nutrient intake and exercise. Optimal management requires an understanding and appreciation of the stresses and burdens of diabetes superimposed on the underlying social and family structure and characteristics.*

In this book, Drs. Michael Harris, Korey Hood, and Jill Weissberg-Benchell, three child psychologists with considerable personal, clinical, and academic experience with children and teenagers with diabetes, use their collective experience to provide a developmental and psychosocial context for optimizing diabetes management in teens. Further, they highlight real-world examples of the conflicts and challenges that exist in adolescents with diabetes and their families and give practical approaches to facilitate resolution. Each chapter tackles a different aspect of adolescent–parent and adolescent–health care provider interactions and uses examples of approaches to deal with the given situation. Health care providers caring for adolescents with type 1 diabetes need to apply these examples and approaches when approaching teenagers with type 1 diabetes and their families.

The first chapter addresses the developmental demands of adolescence and the developmental constructs of why teenagers behave as they do. In the second chapter, the authors address adjustment to the diagnosis of a chronic disease such as diabetes and how diabetes affects the lifestyle of the adolescent. These lifestyle changes are considerable, and it is important that parents and health care providers understand this to maintain a supportive and ongoing relationship.

Chapter 3 addresses the language of diabetes and how what is said and how words are used conveys a message that can be either supportive or obstructive to the interaction and the relationship. Chapter 4 discusses diabetes self-management and the importance of focusing on self-care behaviors and realistic, achievable goals instead of only on unachievable metabolic outcomes. In this context, it is important to note that even with good self-management behaviors, outcomes may not be optimal. Chapter 5 concentrates on the parent-teen relationship and its impact on diabetes. This chapter's primary focus is to highlight the importance of problem-solving strategies and the appropriate distribution of support and responsibility.

The remaining chapters address specific topics that are critical to understanding when working with teens with diabetes. Chapter 6 addresses mood and the risk of distress and depression in teenagers with diabetes. The prevalence of depression is high, and unfavorable consequences on outcomes are frequent. Professional psychological intervention is often necessary. Chapter 7 concentrates on the potential use of new and emerging technologies to benefit teens with diabetes. While the impact of these technologies on the health behaviors of adolescents are not fully known yet, they serve as a promising avenue for optimizing outcomes. Chapters 8 and 9 address important concerns related to repeat diabetic ketoacidosis episodes and high-risk behaviors, respectively. The issues discussed in these chapters include disordered eating and insulin omission, alcohol and other substance abuse, sexual activity, and driving.

Finally, Chapter 10 focuses on the important issue of transition from pediatric to adult health care and Chapter 11 focuses on advocacy—two themes that mark the conclusion of the adolescent period and evolution toward adulthood. These are issues that can fall down on the priority list, since many issues need to be addressed with adolescents; however, they absolutely need to be addressed to set the stage for successful navigation of the adult diabetes world.

Overall, this book provides, through examples based on the experiences of three knowledgeable and very capable clinical psychologists, an evidence-based practical approach to understanding the turmoil inherent in the triad of adolescent, parents, and health care providers. Understanding the developmental state of adolescents and addressing psychosocial, psychoeducational, and family issues that result are critical to providing the best medical care for teens with diabetes and their families. Our success (or failure) as health care providers for youth with diabetes will best be judged by the future success of our patients in their diabetes management and health care as they make the transition to adulthood. In this book, Drs. Harris, Hood, and Weissberg-Benchell lay a framework for these efforts.

Neil H. White, MD, CDE
Professor of Pediatrics
Washington University School of Medicine
St. Louis, Missouri

Acknowledgments

Collectively, we have worked with some of the best diabetes teams across the country, headed up by some of the best endocrinologists. Our work has been heavily influenced by these teams and their physician leaders, including the diabetes teams at St. Louis Children's Hospital in St. Louis, Missouri (Neil H. White, MD, and the late Julio Santiago, MD), Children's National Medical Center in Washington, D.C. (Allen Glasgow, MD, and Fran Cogen, MD), Joslin Diabetes Center in Boston, Massachusetts (Lori Laffel, MD, MPH), Cincinnati Children's Hospital Medical Center in Cincinnati, Ohio (Lawrence Dolan, MD), Lurie Children's Hospital in Chicago, Illinois (Donald Zimmerman, MD), the Harold Schnitzer Diabetes Health Center in Portland, Oregon (Andrew Ahmann, MD, and Bruce Boston, MD), and the Madison Clinic for Pediatric Diabetes in San Francisco, California (Saleh Adi, MD).

In addition, the success of our work has been made possible only through the support, guidance, and direction of the many expert clinicians and scientists in the field of diabetes, including Cindy L. Hanson, PhD, Tim Wysocki, PhD, Barbara J. Anderson, PhD, Richard R. Rubin, PhD, Mark Peyrot, PhD, David Marrero, PhD, Dennis Drotar, PhD, Pat Lustman, PhD, Alan Delamater, PhD, Marilyn Ritholz, PhD, and Suzanne Bennett Johnson, PhD, and the many members of BRIDGE (Behavioral Research in Diabetes Group Exchange).

During the writing of this book, a titan in the field, Dr. Richard R. Rubin, passed away. Dr. Rubin was considered one of the founding fathers of behavioral and psychosocial research in diabetes. He was a key player in many of the large multicenter studies examining better ways to treat diabetes, including the Diabetes Control and Complications Trial (DCCT), the Diabetes Prevention Program (DPP), and Diabetes Attitudes, Wishes, and Needs (DAWN), as well as many others. Along with Dr. Barbara J. Anderson, Dr. Rubin coauthored one of the first books for professionals addressing the psychosocial and behavioral challenges of diabetes care, *Practical Psychology for Diabetes Clinicians* (Anderson and Rubin 1996). Besides being an exemplary researcher and professional, Dr. Rubin was an incredibly grounded and compassionate individual. He was one of the nicest people we have had the pleasure of working with. When speaking about our successes in diabetes, we always think about the expression "standing on the shoulders of giants." Dr. Rubin is and was one of those giants.

We would like to thank our life partners (Ally Burr-Harris, PhD, Neil Benchell, JD, and Diana Naranjo, PhD) for their support, patience, and encouragement throughout our careers. In addition, we would like to thank our own children (Jonah, Solomon, Raechel, Morgan, Maria, Emma, and Naomi) for the valuable lessons they have taught us as parents. They have brought us humility and helped us to "walk the walk," adding to our ability to keep it real in our professional work with adolescents.

Finally, we would like to thank all the families of teens with diabetes whom we have worked with over the years. We are continually amazed at how they cope with the complexity of diabetes on top of the complexity of adolescence. Although all three of us have been trained in psychology, child development, and diabetes, most of what we have learned has come from our direct work with hundreds of teens with diabetes and their families. We are forever indebted to these remarkable young people and their equally remarkable families.

Introduction

Teens with diabetes pose unique challenges for professionals working in diabetes care. Possible challenges range from the teen diagnosed with diabetes as a child who was previously a model patient and now struggles with his or her diabetes care, to a young person diagnosed with diabetes during adolescence who is struggling to integrate diabetes care into the "normal" life of a teen. We have found that many well-intending health care professionals fall back on the old strategy of "scared straight" as a means of trying to get teens to take better care of their diabetes. In essence, the scared straight approach involves lecturing teens about the likely long-term consequences of not taking care of their diabetes, including retinopathy, gangrene, and kidney failure. Yet we know that teens often are living in the now and are less worried about potential consequences down the road than adults.

The other common strategy we have observed many health care professionals using is to shift the focus to the parents and encourage them to take control of their teen's diabetes care. Unfortunately, this approach, as most developmental psychologists know, is counter to the developmental demands of adolescence. To ask teens to accept parental control over domains they had previously controlled is akin to getting your driver's license and then being told you cannot drive. This strategy is doomed to fail because most teens are seeking greater independence from their parents and are not receptive to handing control back to them. Any attempts by parents to take the control back are met with a high degree of resistance. A confluence of normal development, a complex medical condition, and frustrated professionals creates a perfect storm. The teens with diabetes and their families are unhappy, and the professionals working with teens with diabetes are frustrated. Ultimately, the aforementioned scenario results in poorer diabetes self-management and poorer metabolic control for teens with diabetes. Thus, we have written this book to address this very challenging population in hopes of improving care delivered to teens with diabetes and, in turn, improving the health behaviors and health status of teens with diabetes.

Collectively, our experiences with families of teens with diabetes have taught us valuable lessons. In this book, we provide professionals with a developmental framework for a better understanding of the normal developmental demands of adolescence and how those normal developmental demands may impact the management of diabetes during adolescence. Within this developmental framework, we also provide strategies for negotiating the many challenges of providing care to teens with diabetes. We identify common teenage issues (e.g., sexuality, smoking, drugs/alcohol, and depression) and discuss how they can be exacerbated by diabetes. Finally, we review subjects specific to teens with diabetes, such as insulin pumps, continuous glucose monitors, diabetes advocacy, and the transition from pediatric to adult diabetes care.

In each chapter we provide an overview of the interactions between development, diabetes, and family. We present case examples to further elucidate the issues, and then we provide suggestions for both assessment and intervention. This book is best used as a reference guide for professionals working with teens with diabetes and their families. Although some of the topics are unique to current approaches to diabetes management (e.g., technology and diabetes care), the bulk of the information provided is timeless and applicable to adolescents dealing with other complex medical conditions.

Michael A. Harris, PhD
Harold Schnitzer Diabetes
    Health Center
Oregon Health & Science University
Portland, Oregon

Jill Weissberg-Benchell, PhD, CDE
Lurie Children's Hospital
Northwestern University
Chicago, Illinois

Korey K. Hood, PhD
Madison Clinic for Pediatric Diabetes
University of California, San Francisco
San Francisco, California

1
Developmental Demands of Adolescence

If you work with teenagers or they live in your home, you are well aware of their many great qualities. Teenagers are eager to grow up and have new experiences, and have a sense of invincibility mixed with some innocence and naïveté. Your experience with teenagers has also led you to understand their rapidly fluctuating emotions, brazen attitudes, and, at times, difficulty appreciating the importance of taking care of themselves. This chapter will provide a context for why teenagers behave the way they do and how different approaches may be necessary when interacting with teenagers. This chapter will help you when that next adolescent patient shows up in your clinic and displays a defiance of convention, a preference for social priorities over personal priorities, and a sense of invulnerability and invincibility. We also discuss how these adolescent qualities affect diabetes management.

Developmental Context

More than 100 years ago, the child development pioneer G. Stanley Hall described adolescence as a time of "storm and stress." According to Hall (1904), adolescence is marked by three major changes: emotional upheaval, increased risk taking, and extreme parent-child conflict. Hall believed that this period of development is biologically driven and largely universal, but especially problematic for adolescents in the U.S. Hall cited urbanization and individualism as additional causes of storm and stress in U.S. adolescents.

Since Hall's initial description of adolescence, others have examined the concept of storm and stress empirically. An American psychologist, Jeffrey Arnett (1999), examined adolescents and young adults and coined the term emerging adult, which will be discussed later in the context of transition. In contrast to Hall's idea of an across-the-board tumultuous time specific to adolescence, Arnett found that rates of psychopathology were relatively consistent from childhood into adolescence and that most youth were not experiencing significant psychological distress. Further, there was no major shift in risk taking during adolescence; however, the consequences of the risks taken by adolescents were much greater than the risks taken by children. Finally, Arnett concurred with Hall in confirming an increase in parent-child conflict as children mature into adolescents.

Arnett's debunking of Hall's assertion that adolescence is universally a time of storm and stress, paired with the evidence of unique challenges across biologic, physiologic, and cognitive developments for adolescents, leads to the following assumptions:

- Most adolescent patients do not experience profound psychological distress, but instead experience the normal demands of navigating this developmental period.
- Most adolescent patients do not intend to be "difficult."
- You should approach each encounter with an adolescent patient with a fresh perspective, because development will trigger almost daily changes in attitudes, perceptions, and mood.

Further, to be fully prepared to help the adolescent patient in front of you, consider the areas discussed below.

Defiance of Convention

When working with adolescents, most professionals struggle with the normal developmental demand of defiance of convention. Defiance of convention is characterized by pushing against the status quo and challenging authority as a means of developing a sense of self. Teens are trying on a number of personality "hats" to define who they are and how they are different from parents and teachers. Besides parents and teachers, health care providers also represent convention. So when teens do not follow the directives of health care providers, they are doing what one would expect developmentally. The single best example of this is the "Just Say No" campaign for which former first lady Nancy Reagan was the spokesperson. Data on the effectiveness of the "Just Say No" campaign and other similarly messaged campaigns indicate that authority figures used for campaigns targeting teens are of questionable effectiveness (Fishbein 2002). Few represent convention and authority more than the wife of the president of the United States.

"I Wonder If She Likes Me?"

Teens are generally more focused on their social relationships than on their families. Much of social and moral learning comes from peers rather than parents, which is a shift from childhood, when parents were more influential. Data show that although there is some increase in parent-teen conflict during adolescence, parents can and should remain an important influence in the teen's life. This influence is different from the influence parents have with younger children. With younger children, it is the spoken message of the parent that affects them. However, with teens, it is the parents' behavior rather than what they say that carries the most weight. Parents often continue to try to "talk some sense" into their teens, as do professionals. It often seems like the teens only hear "wah, wah, wah," as depicted when adults talk in Charlie Brown cartoons. Professionals may not realize that their reminders and lectures (though perhaps necessary) do not have the same impact on a teen as they have on a younger child.

In the realm of diabetes care, parents and professionals may conclude that teens do not care about their diabetes. The truth is that teens do care about their diabetes, but there are competing demands that hold a higher level of priority in a teen's life. Instead of giving instructions and offering advice, the professional might ask if there are other areas that are creating stress and making it hard to manage diabetes, or offer suggestions in those areas in an attempt to alleviate stress and make more time for diabetes management. For example, parents and teens are likely to be embroiled in conflict over curfew, homework, or chores. If a professional were able to offer suggestions about non–diabetes-related conflicts, then the parents and their teens might have more time to focus on diabetes management. The most successful suggestions from professionals should involve a quid pro quo solution where both parents and teens are giving something to get something.

Invulnerability and Invincibility

Developmentally, teens do not have the cognitive capacity to fully understand how their actions today will impact their lives in the future, especially when it comes to thinking about their own mortality. Parents (and health care providers) want teens with diabetes to see how their health behaviors today will impact their lives in the future. It is not uncommon for health care providers and parents to resort to the scared straight approach with teens around their health. For example, health care providers might take teens with diabetes to a dialysis unit to show them what will happen in the event that they evidence kidney disease from poorly controlled diabetes. Developmentally, most teens are unaffected by this and often are more impressed with the technology and science of dialysis. The scared straight approach has been implemented in many areas, including juvenile justice, but has shown little effect on behavior (Ashton 1999, Lilenfeld 2005). If teens could understand how their behaviors today will impact their health in the future, they would not be teens—they would be adults. The ability to change current behavior to avoid negative long-term consequences depends in part on the maturity of brain development, a process that is not completed until adulthood. This brain development is not magically sped up when young people are diagnosed with diabetes such that they suddenly make the link between current behavior and future outcomes.

What *does* happen to all children as they mature into teens, however, is that they begin to naturally question authority as they develop the cognitive skill of abstract reasoning. Teens begin to see the disconnect between what they are told by adults and authority figures, and what they see adults and authority figures do. For example, a teen with diabetes is being lectured about needing to take better care of his or her health (through more exercise, better eating habits, etc.), but is trying to reconcile that message coming from parents, health care providers, and other adults who do not exercise or eat well.

How Does Adolescence Affect Diabetes Management?

It is well established that the teen years are the most difficult time to control blood glucose levels. Although the reasons for this trend are multifaceted and complex, we do know that adolescence is the time when diabetes self-management is the poorest. We also know that dramatic changes in one's body have a negative impact on blood glucose levels, and clearly adolescence is a time of major physical maturation. Many professionals continue to view diabetes control as a proxy for adherence in diabetes. However, research has shown that there is not a one-to-one relationship between health behaviors and diabetes control in diabetes (i.e., the hemoglobin A1C value). There are many other factors that can impact blood glucose levels, including development, stress, and the natural course of diabetes. Focusing on diabetes control as the primary outcome for teens with diabetes is a setup for failure for both the teens and the health care providers.

Instead of focusing on diabetes control in teens with diabetes, focus on health behaviors. These behaviors include checking blood glucose values, taking insulin, and counting carbohydrates. These are things that teens have control over and that can produce immediate and visible improvements. Likewise, although there is not a one-to-one relationship between health behaviors and diabetes control, there is evidence that as health behaviors improve, diabetes control will likely also improve. For example, a simple change like helping a teen to take his or her insulin before rather than after he or she eats will undoubtedly have a positive impact on diabetes control because blood glucose levels will not immediately spike during a meal.

Case Example

Casey is a 16-year-old male diagnosed with diabetes when he was 4 years old. Casey lives with his parents, 14-year-old sister, 10-year-old sister, and 5-year-old twin brothers. Both of Casey's parents work and are college educated. Casey's diabetes control has been quite good, with A1C values in the mid-7% range until recently. Casey's diabetes self-management was always at the highest level and he has always been able to manage his diabetes independently when at school or away from home. Within the past 2 years, Casey's A1C values have averaged around 9%, and he frequently reports forgetting to bolus at lunch. Casey has frequently gone to high school sporting events without his insulin and has eaten while at these events without bolusing. Casey's parents are very upset with him for not caring about his diabetes, taking huge risks with his health, and not being aware of how his current diabetes self-management will impact his diabetes down the road. Casey's parents have decided to take back the control for his diabetes and not allow him to spend time with friends or go out on weekends and evenings until his diabetes control has improved.

In addition, Casey's parents have not allowed him to sign up for driver's education and will not allow him to do so until his diabetes control has improved. Casey has been referred to the clinic psychologist by his parents to address the problem of "his not caring about his diabetes."

Assessment and Intervention

This is a typical case in that Casey and his parents begin to struggle as he matures from being a child with diabetes into being an adolescent with diabetes. Developmentally, Casey is attending to the priority of most teens, his social relationships. Likewise, Casey's parents are viewing the changes in Casey's behavior through the lens of storm and stress and responding reflexively with attempts at taking back the control. In this particular case, the intervention could be something as simple as psychoeducation around normal adolescent development, thus providing insight to Casey's parents about his change in behavior. Casey could also benefit from a discussion about how to attend simultaneously to his desire to be a "normal teenager" and to the demands of his diabetes. The intervention for Casey involved the aforementioned along with moving him off insulin shots and onto an insulin pump. This allowed Casey greater freedom to come and go as he pleased, while having his insulin with him at all times to accommodate impromptu changes in his activities and eating.

2
Adjustment to Diagnosis During Adolescence

Being diagnosed with diabetes during adolescence can be a very difficult challenge at an already stressful time of development. Children diagnosed with diabetes at a young age often do not remember a life without diabetes once they reach adolescence. The years of a familiar diabetes care routine can be a protective factor for many teens. However, when a young person has lived 13 or more years without diabetes and then is told he or she has diabetes, the adjustment can be quite difficult. The diagnosis brings with it significant lifestyle changes.

Although teens are better prepared cognitively than children to manage diabetes, given their stronger abstract reasoning and higher cognitive-processing abilities, the shift away from tight parental supervision and monitoring leaves them vulnerable to poor diabetes self-care. Compared to children, teens are more in control of what they eat and what they are doing when away from their homes, and they have established some pretty strong patterns around health behaviors such as exercise and diet. Teens live much less structured lives compared to their younger counterparts. During adolescence, sleep patterns are known to shift dramatically, eating patterns often change markedly, and reliance on parents rapidly decreases. Unfortunately, it is well established that living a more structured life makes diabetes management easier, given that many of the diabetes management tasks happen around regular meals and during the waking hours of the day. If a teen is used to eating whenever he or she wants and goes to sleep late at night and wakes up in the afternoon on weekends, diabetes care becomes more of a challenge.

Because teens have more sophisticated cognitive-processing skills than children, they can more readily establish a causal relationship between their health behaviors and health outcomes. While still in the hospital at diagnosis, teens begin to establish a strong connection between the food they eat, the insulin they take, and their blood glucose levels. Within hours of a teen's first reading, he or she will begin to pair diabetes-specific tasks with achieving a blood glucose number in the target range. This is an adaptive behavior that gives teens control over a situation in which they feel completely out of control. Making a direct connection between engaging in self-care tasks and keeping blood glucose levels in the target zone simplifies what is being asked of adolescents. "If I check my blood glucose levels and calculate my carbs and insulin, then I will be fine," they think. Unfortunately, diabetes care is not that simple, and there is not a one-to-one relationship between metabolic control and health behaviors. Then teens begin to view diabetes management as a game that, if played correctly, they can win. However, as soon as a teen has a blood glucose level out of the target range, he or she thinks of that as a loss in the diabetes game or a "bad" thing. Likewise, when the teen has a blood glucose level in the target range, he or she thinks of that as a win or a "good" thing. When blood glucose levels are viewed as good and bad, teens begin to view themselves as doing well or badly at managing diabetes, and then quickly make the jump to "I am good or I am bad based on what my blood glucose level is." Unfortunately, given the nature of diabetes, teens have more blood glucose levels out of target than in target... *a lot of bad and not much good.* Teens may not let their disproportionate number of "bad" blood glucose readings prevent them from taking care of their diabetes; they may instead solve the problem by not checking their blood glucose levels, to avoid being reminded of all the bad. So although they may get their insulin, these teens are making guesses about amounts of insulin that are based on guesses about blood glucose levels. This is clearly not a way to successfully manage one's diabetes.

Although this maladaptive thinking pattern about good/bad blood glucose numbers is something we see clinically on a daily basis, it can be prevented by health care professionals. We recommend that health care professionals discuss the reality of blood glucose variability with adolescent patients and their parents. The fact that variables we cannot measure (e.g., pubertal hormones, stress) impact blood glucose outcomes needs to be discussed. Moreover, we recommend focusing on adolescents' self-care behaviors (e.g., checking blood glucose levels, counting carbohydrates, bolusing before meals) more than on the blood glucose outcomes. When adolescents focus on engaging in self-care behaviors and also focus on fixing out-of-range numbers instead of feeling worried, guilty, or demoralized about out-of-range numbers, their metabolic and psychosocial outcomes improve.

Another challenge that teens newly diagnosed with diabetes have is the bigger-picture question: "What does this mean for me and the rest of my life?" A younger child diagnosed with diabetes is quick to view his or her diabetes as a temporary thing, and so to some degree that type of thinking is adaptive in getting the child to "temporarily" make all the changes necessary to accommodate diabetes care. However, teens newly diagnosed with diabetes have the ability to understand that their diabetes is not a temporary condition and that they will likely have to take care of their diabetes for the rest of their lives. This realization can quickly overwhelm a teen at diagnosis and make it difficult to see a life with diabetes that is "normal" and in which he or she can experience success (e.g., college, career, marriage).

Finally, we see parents of teens newly diagnosed with diabetes struggling to know how best to parent, either around the diabetes management or around typical parent-teen issues. Parents typically do one of two things when their teenager is diagnosed with diabetes. Some parents view diabetes as a sickness and begin to back off on typical expectations they may have had of their child. These parents are quick to allow their children to skip school when not feeling well, to drop out of normal activities (e.g., sports, clubs) for fear of low blood glucose, and to avoid spending time away from home (e.g., sleeping over with friends, going to the beach). Other parents view the challenge of diabetes management as a cognitive and behavioral exercise that teens are capable of doing independently. These parents are quick to assume that once properly educated, their teen can and should take care of his or her diabetes without any assistance. These parents forget that a newly diagnosed teen faces enormous psychological, social, and emotional challenges that can have an impact on the success of diabetes self-management.

Case Example

Abby is a previously healthy 14-year-old female who was diagnosed with diabetes during a hospitalization after 2 weeks of frequent urination, increased thirst, increased appetite, and frequent fatigue, and weight loss of about 15 lb over the past month. Abby currently lives with her mother and 17-year-old brother. She visits with her father weekly. Abby just began high school and is an active person. She participates in softball, basketball, and volleyball. Abby is an excellent student and has many friends. With all of her activities, Abby has a very unstructured life. Sometimes she is home from school at 4:00 p.m., while other times she is not home until 8:00 p.m. or 9:00 p.m. because of a late game or practice. Abby is frequently up late doing homework, and on school nights does not get to bed until 11:00 p.m. or midnight. Weekends are equally inconsistent. Some weekends Abby sleeps in until noon and other weekends she is up earlier for practices or games. At diagnosis, Abby appeared largely unaffected by the challenges of managing her diabetes, and her mother also never appeared worried about Abby's ability to successfully manage her diabetes. Abby was viewed by the medical team as a model patient and mature beyond her years. At times during diabetes education, Abby appeared to be competing with her mother over diabetes knowledge and the "right" thing to say when asked about carbohydrate counting, insulin adjustment, and blood glucose checking.

Assessment and Intervention

An initial assessment of Abby might lead one to think that she is well on her way to successfully adjusting to and managing her diabetes. However, several things stand out as possible problems that might cause Abby to struggle with her diabetes after she is discharged from the hospital. The primary issue that might trip up Abby is also an asset in other situations; that is, being so bright and excelling academically. Understanding what one needs to do is not enough for successful management of diabetes. In Abby's case, this conundrum is compounded by the fact that her mother sees her as competent and capable without considering the other critical psychological, social, and emotional factors that go into successful diabetes management. Without some intervention, Abby and her mother would be headed home with the presumption that Abby can take care of her diabetes independently. Another issue that might be easily overlooked is Abby's competitive nature and her focus on getting it right. This could quickly lead to discouragement and frustration when Abby is doing every-thing right, but her blood glucose levels are not in the target range. What we often see with such young people is that they intensify their diabe-tes self-management efforts and then eventually burn out because those efforts are not sustainable alongside the busy schedule of a teen athlete. Finally, it is clear that Abby's lifestyle will present challenges to success-ful diabetes management. Abby's irregular sleep and eating schedules will make it difficult to establish patterns in managing her diabetes.

Treatment for Abby would involve a conversation with her and her mother about the need to work together in managing Abby's diabetes. We tell families that no matter how smart, how experienced, or how old some-one is, we don't see anyone managing diabetes successfully alone. We talk with families about the goal being "interdependence" around diabe-tes management, not "independence": "interdependence" being defined as the use of friends and family to help and support diabetes manage-ment. The goal is for Abby to be maximally independent in daily life and minimally burdened by diabetes. Treatment would also involve a discus-sion of the concept that blood glucose levels are neither good nor bad. Instead, all blood glucose levels should be viewed as good and as valu-able bits of information to help guide Abby, her mother, and the medical team in good diabetes care. This strategy also allows for disentanglement of Abby's blood glucose levels and her actual diabetes care behaviors. In other words, we would help Abby understand that because of other factors out of her control, she will likely have high and low blood glucose numbers despite optimal diabetes self-management.

3
Language of Diabetes

Psycholinguistics is the psychology of language. The language that we use has a huge impact on our own behavior as well as the behavior of others. There is no better example of this than the self-fulfilling prophecy, where what we tell ourselves about a situation oftentimes becomes our destiny (Merton 1968). If you tell yourself that you will be unhappy with something, it is likely that you will, in fact, be unhappy. This is not to say that our thoughts and beliefs automatically become reality, but we tend to focus on and remember aspects of our experiences that confirm what we already believe and feel to be the case. We tend to dismiss or ignore evidence that contradicts those beliefs. Psychologists call this the confirmation bias (Nickerson 1998). We see this process set in motion very early on in the life of someone with diabetes. Those who learn to think about making the best of their diabetes and not to hate having diabetes are more likely to cope with the natural struggles of having this chronic health condition, while those who think their lives are ruined because of diabetes will find confirmatory evidence. Clearly, health care professionals working with teens with diabetes should be mindful of how they talk about diabetes.

In addition, the language that professionals use with patients has been linked to health outcomes (Street 2009). For example, a systematic review of studies examining the outcomes of communication interventions targeting physician–patient encounters found that, generally, communication interventions led to more productive physician–patient encounters and in many of the studies improved health outcomes (Griffin 2004).

Obviously, teens are very sensitive to the words that we use, and in many cases we use strong language with teens that does not truly reflect the reality of the situation. A simple example that many parents and professionals use is the statement: "You need to take more responsibility for your diabetes." Cloaked in that statement is the belief that the teen is being irresponsible about his or her diabetes and/or doesn't take it seriously enough. The ultimate misuse of language with teens with diabetes—or with anyone who has a chronic health condition—is to say they are *noncompliant*. To say that a patient is noncompliant is factually incorrect, as collectively we have never met any teen with diabetes who is noncompliant. His or her compliance may be less than stellar, but the teen is never totally noncompliant. This phrasing allows for only two options, compliant or noncompliant, perpetuating the myth that there is only one right way to manage this complicated and ever-changing disease. The research suggests that only about 7% of individuals with diabetes are fully compliant with their treatment regimen at any given time (i.e., doing every diabetes-related task expected of them at exactly the time it is expected to be done). The second way that the use of the word *compliance* is a problem is that *noncompliance* is a term that suggests children are purposefully ignoring the directives of a parent, perpetuating a paternalistic model of care. The fact that the word is pejorative only makes matters worse. Although the term *noncompliance* has been and still is used by well-meaning health care providers, it does not provide the information necessary for high-quality care that encourages shared decision making. With this judgmental frame of reference, where does one start in terms of providing medical care to a teen with diabetes?

The Society of Pediatric Psychology chose not to use the term *noncompliance* in any of its publications because of its pejorative connotation. More recently, many health care providers have switched over from describing patients as *noncompliant* to describing them as *nonadherent*. Although the use of the term *nonadherence* is less condescending, it still limits communication about the patient's health behaviors in that it frames behavior around complex tasks as dichotomous: patients are either adherent or nonadherent. The use of both nonadherence and noncompliance significantly limits effective communication with patients about their health behaviors. Given that most medical care is based on patient self-report, the full picture is not realized when using the terms *compliance* or *adherence* with patients, especially teen patients. Instead of using these words, facilitate effective communication with patients by asking them how they are doing managing their diabetes. This allows for questions about times and conditions when they are able to do what is being asked of them, as well as when they struggle with their treatment regimen.

Example: Paternalistic Language

Physician: Have you been compliant with your diabetes regimen?

    Teen: Yes.

Physician: So you're getting all your insulin and testing your blood glucose five times per day as I asked you to do?

    Teen: Yes.

Example: Collaborative Language

Physician: So, my guess is, like most people with diabetes, you are pretty good at some parts of your diabetes management, while other things are harder to do or to remember to do. Tell me, what is going well with your diabetes self-management?

    Teen: I always remember to take my Lantus and I'm good about counting carbs.

Physician: Excellent. How are you able to remember to take your Lantus all the time?

    Teen: It's actually pretty easy because I take my Lantus in the evening and since I am getting ready for bed it has just become a routine.

Physician: What is harder for you to do?

    Teen: Well, I don't always remember to take my Humalog at lunch because I don't want to go to the office when everyone else is eating.

Two more words that imply purposeful, mean-spirited behavioral choices are sneaking and cheating. Parents frequently report that their teen is sneaking food or cheating on a meal plan or eating the "wrong foods." What we ask parents in these situations is, "Since when does eating food become sneaking or cheating? When did eating food become a clandestine activity?" In addition, using these terms with teens turns the eating of food into a cat-and-mouse game between parents and their teens. The more that a teen feels he or she is doing something wrong, the better he or she gets at hiding it. Knowing what someone is eating is critical for proper diabetes care so that proper adjustments can be made in insulin. Therefore, it is vital to set the stage for open communication and problem solving about eating choices, instead of creating an environment where the goal is avoiding conversations with parents.

Many years ago, before the advent of short-acting insulin such as Novalog or Humalog, the consumption of simple sugars was discouraged. However, with short-acting insulin, people with diabetes are now able to eat as they wish and minimize a spike in blood glucose. Clearly, whether or not you have diabetes, moderate consumption of most types of foods is the way to go. However, many teens feel punished for having diabetes, and restricting what types of food they can or should eat will contribute to a backlash, with the teens eating more of the foods we would encourage them to limit and/or not telling anyone what they are really eating.

Many health care providers, as well as parents of teens with diabetes, say that teens don't care about their diabetes. As with many of the other things that are said about teens with diabetes, this statement is factually inaccurate. Not caring *about* one's diabetes would translate into not doing anything to care *for* one's diabetes, such as not taking any insulin, never checking blood glucose levels, eating whatever and whenever, and never obtaining medical care for diabetes. This just doesn't happen in diabetes. What does happen is that teens don't adhere at the level that medical providers and parents would like them to. Instead of five or seven blood glucose checks per day, a teen may be checking his or her blood glucose five or seven times per week or per month. This reflects less-than-optimal self-care, but it also reflects an effort on the teen's part to care for his or her diabetes. This may seem insignificant to most health care professionals working with this population; however, any self-care effort represents an opportunity to reinforce a teen for doing the right thing. Most interactions between health care professionals and teens with diabetes are void of anything positive unless the teen's metabolic control is in the 7% range, which is unlikely.

Reinforcing a teen for even showing up to clinic represents a move in the right direction and provides leverage for improvements in health behaviors. As one of our beloved colleagues (Dr. Richard R. Rubin) often said, there is only one acceptable response when a person checks blood glucose (regardless of the number on the meter at the time): "Thank you for checking." It is the behavior of checking that we want to reinforce, as such acknowledgement increases the chance of that person checking again.

Having a patient take sole responsibility for diabetes should not be a goal of any diabetes clinic, regardless of the age of the patient. Yet providers and parents often talk about the need for teens to "take responsibility" for their diabetes. What does this mean? In most cases, it means that teens should do all that is necessary for optimal diabetes care completely by themselves without anyone reminding them of what they need to do. Because teens are sensitive to the words we use, the need to "take responsibility for diabetes" is heard as "You are irresponsible." Teens lose their house keys, forget homework assignments, oversleep, etc. Why would anyone expect them to treat diabetes-related tasks differently than other tasks?

Diabetes self-care is best illustrated by first thinking of those without diabetes as having a movie going on inside their bodies where all the organs know the plot and make changes without any input or effort on the part of the person. In contrast, those with diabetes only get four or five still photographs of what is going on inside their bodies, and they must now guess the plot and make adjustments from outside their bodies. If you think of it this way, it's quite amazing that our patients do as well as they do, especially our adolescent patients. So trying to get teens with diabetes to take on more responsibility for managing their diabetes is unrealistic, unfair, and likely to be doomed as a means of improving self-care behaviors.

Finally, many people still use the word diabetic when referring to patients or when referring to themselves. Most teens with diabetes are struggling not to be diabetic, and instead are trying to be teens (with diabetes). Using the term *diabetic* does not do justice to the person as a whole and reduces his or her existence down to a medical condition. Many people refer to themselves as diabetic, which is their right. However, avoiding the term *diabetic* when treating teens with diabetes helps to remind everyone (yourself, other professionals, parents, and patients) that diabetes is just one part of a teen's life and doesn't define who he or she is. One concrete way you can focus on the whole person (as opposed to pancreatic function) is to start each clinic visit with a conversation about an aspect of your patient's life that has nothing to do with blood glucose: "How did that soccer championship go?" "How did that paper you were working on turn out?" "How was homecoming?" "What are your summer plans?"

Case Example

Kelly is a 13-year-old female with diabetes. Kelly was diagnosed with diabetes when she was 9 years old. She has been hospitalized four times for diabetic ketoacidosis (DKA) since her diagnosis, with two times being in the past 6 months. Kelly's metabolic control has typically been in the 9% range; however, in the past 2 years her A1C values have consistently been around 13%. Kelly lives with her mother, stepfather, and 17-year-old brother. Kelly is in the seventh grade and is an average student. She is active in drama, dance, and choir. Kelly's biological father lives out of state and she spends summers with him. Kelly's biological father has type 1 diabetes and is sympathetic to Kelly's struggles with her diabetes. Kelly's stepfather is obese and has type 2 diabetes. In clinic, Kelly's mother and stepfather frequently berate her in front of the health care team for lying about her blood glucose checks, sneaking food, and not taking responsibility for her diabetes. Kelly's stepfather believes that Kelly doesn't care about her diabetes and as a result will most certainly be on dialysis before she is 20 years old. During her clinic visits, Kelly vacillates between defending herself to her parents and becoming tearful. Kelly is referred to as a noncompliant patient and a "train wreck" by her endocrinologist. Kelly is steadfast in her denial about mismanaging her diabetes and reports that she hates having diabetes.

Assessment and Intervention

Clearly, Kelly and her family are buried under a mound of negative language about her diabetes. In addition, Kelly's own language about her diabetes is negative (i.e., "I hate having diabetes."). Kelly and her family need some psychoeducation about the power of language and how they talk about her and her diabetes. In addition, it would be important to challenge Kelly's mother and stepfather on their assumptions that Kelly doesn't care about her health or about taking care of her diabetes.

A good strategy to use in these situations is to challenge parents to think about what a teen gets out of not caring for himself/herself. If they struggle with this, you can point out that a teen like Kelly gets to deal with upset parents, disappointed doctors and nurses, highly conflictual clinic visits, and, frequently, high blood glucose levels that make her feel sick. Tackling the linked issues of "not being responsible" and being destined for bad outcomes is very important for Kelly and her family. This language is a setup for Kelly because no matter what she does to take better care of her diabetes, her parents seem convinced that she is doomed to failure. The most effective strategy in this case would be to remind Kelly's parents that most kids and teens live in the here and now; any discussion of the future is not something that most teens consider. Kelly's parents obviously want to help her to take better care of her diabetes, but have resorted to what many parents fall back on: scare tactics and negative language. Professionals can highlight that Kelly's parents are not angry. Rather, they are worried about her and her diabetes and don't know how to help her. Professionals can explain that the use of scare tactics and negative language is driven by concern and love, and this may help both the parents and the teen to see things differently.

Once the reason that the parents are being so negative with Kelly is reframed, professionals can highlight that the parents' strategy is not working. Kelly's parents need to acknowledge that another approach is warranted. Kelly and her parents need coaching in order to talk about diabetes in both neutral and more positive language that has a better chance of helping Kelly think differently about her diabetes and, in turn, improve her diabetes self-management.

4
Diabetes Self-Management

When teens resist proper diabetes care, they can become consumed with diabetes in a way that further exacerbates their health. This is best understood using quicksand and the Chinese finger trap as analogies. In the example of quicksand, the more one struggles to get out, the more one is pulled down into the quicksand. Experts in quicksand tell people not to struggle and instead to try to lie flat, which will allow the body to slowly get released from the powerful suction of the sand. In the case of the Chinese finger trap, once your fingers go in, the harder you try to pull out, the tighter the trap gets around your fingers. Like getting out of quicksand, getting out of a Chinese finger trap involves relaxing your fingers and slowly pulling them out.

Diabetes presents a similar challenge: the more people fight and resist diabetes, the stronger the hold diabetes has on them. This struggle can be accentuated during adolescence, as young people with diabetes resist parent involvement, seeing it as intrusive, controlling, and distrustful. So when a parent is trying to remain involved in his or her teen's diabetes care by reminding them about taking insulin or checking blood glucose, the teen is hearing nothing but nagging from his or her parent. This escalates into the teen retreating further from his or her parents and the parents pushing harder and harder to remain involved in their teen's diabetes management. Like the quicksand and Chinese finger trap analogies, this just tightens the grip that diabetes has on both the teen and his or her parents.

Many teens with diabetes are overwhelmed by the demands of diabetes care alongside their effort to live a normal life of a teenager. The long slog of diabetes self-management for teens results in shortcuts and less-than-optimal care that may not have immediate consequences, but will likely affect their health over the long term. For example, we find that many teens are quick to size up their meals in terms of carbohydrates and then shoot their insulin based on how they feel and how much they think they will be eating. What they are skipping are blood glucose checks, which can be critical to dosing the right amount of insulin. These teens stay out of DKA, but run A1C values that are less than optimal.

Another common practice for teens with diabetes is waiting to take their insulin until after they eat rather than before. Because teens consume highly variable amounts of food on irregular eating schedules, they are frequently uncertain about how much they will eat at a given meal and likely want to avoid giving more insulin than they might need. They see taking their insulin after the meal as a way of avoiding a low blood glucose level. The obvious problem with giving insulin after a meal is that the blood glucose level has likely already spiked, which is something that should be avoided (i.e., frequent high and low blood glucose levels). As with skipping blood glucose checks, taking insulin after eating typically does not result in any short-term consequences such as DKA, but does affect diabetes longer-term.

Another challenge of diabetes self-management involves the battle between the "wants" in the moment versus the "shoulds" that come after self-reflection. In his book *The Happiness Hypothesis,* Jonathan Haidt (2006) writes about how many, if not all, of our decisions are driven largely by emotion. Haidt cleverly describes the decision-making process as a rider on an elephant, the rider being our rational brain and the elephant being our emotional brain. We like to think that the decisions we make as adults are "rational, based on objective data, and driven by logic and reason" (Haidt 2006). However, even with adults, most decisions are heavily influenced by emotional states. For example, we are on a diet and it is late at night and we are watching television. A commercial comes on for ice cream. We immediately engage our rational brain and tell ourselves that ice cream is not on our diet plan. However, we have had a long day and we have been engaging the rider throughout the day to overcome the desires of the elephant. Our rational brain is exhausted and our elephant heads for the freezer, where we have a pint of ice cream. While we are walking to the freezer, our rational brain continues in a faint voice to remind us of our commitment to our diet. Eventually, the elephant wins over and we consume the entire pint of ice cream.

We see the same struggle in teens with diabetes around self-management tasks. The teen knows he or she needs to take insulin and has every intention of doing so, but as it gets closer and closer to the time for his or her insulin, the desires of the teen's emotional brain take the lead and guide him or her to something less rational and more enjoyable.

Case Example

Jake is a 15-year-old male with diabetes who was diagnosed when he was 11 months old. Jake is an only child. Both of Jake's parents are physicians. Jake's mother is a cardiologist and his father is a general internist. Jake's diabetes self-management has fluctuated. At times, Jake has been able to successfully manage his diabetes; at other times he has struggled. The only time Jake has ever been hospitalized for DKA was when he was diagnosed. However, within the past 6 years Jake's metabolic control has been less than optimal, with A1C values ranging from 9% to 12%. Jake reported that he doesn't need to count carbs because he knows his diabetes so well that he can size things up quickly and determine approximately how many carbs he will be eating and how much insulin he will need. Jake has gotten in the habit of taking his insulin after he eats, as he is very concerned about the social implications of evidencing a low when he is with his friends. Although he reportedly checks his blood glucose three to four times a day, Jake feels this is unnecessary because he believes he can tell what his blood glucose is, based on how he feels. Because Jake has multiple blood glucose meters (one at home, one at school, one in the car), there is no way to determine how many times he is actually checking his blood glucose. Jake is solely responsible for his diabetes management and regards any attempts by his parents to help as nagging. Jake's parents believe that he really doesn't care about his diabetes.

Assessment and Intervention

Given that one of the developmental demands of adolescence is the shift in power and control from parents to the adolescent, using a concrete business model can help Jake and his parents make this shift. Presenting Jake and his parents with the "CEO (Chief Executive Officer) Model of Diabetes Management" appropriately puts Jake in the driver's seat and maintains parental involvement in diabetes care. Jake and his parents are presented with the keys to successful businesses, which include having a CEO who hires good employees, delegates tasks to the employees, and gives regular accurate feedback to the employees about how the company is doing. In the case of teens with diabetes like Jake, they represent the CEOs. Their company is diabetes. Unfortunately, they cannot sell the company. The company will be theirs until there is a cure for diabetes. However, the company can be successful with the aforementioned ingredients. Who are the employees for teens with diabetes? Doctors, certified diabetes educators (CDEs), psychologists, medical social workers, parents, older siblings, friends, extended family, coaches, teachers, and other important people in the teen's life. The next step is to put Jake's employees to work on helping the company succeed. Successful companies do not have CEOs doing all the work, nor do they have CEOs who go into their offices and tell all the employees to leave them alone. This is the hard part, as teens love to be in charge, but struggle to tell others what they need from them. Teens know what they don't want (e.g., "don't nag me, don't ask me if I took my insulin"), but don't know what would help them better care for their diabetes. Finally, to ensure that problems are being identified and resolved earlier rather than later, Jake needs to regularly and accurately provide feedback and information to his health care providers and parents (key employees) on how his diabetes is going. Since most diabetes care is based on self-report coupled with metabolic control, having accurate information about how, when, and under what conditions Jake is giving himself insulin is critical to making any adjustments to improve health outcomes.

Although goal setting is one of the most basic and effective tools that health care professionals have at their disposal in helping people better manage their health, few use this strategy with their patients. The first key to successful goal setting is knowing what the patient's true baseline is for any given behavior. In Jake's case, knowing how many times he is actually checking his blood glucose allows for setting an achievable goal. For example, if Jake is only checking one time per week, but everyone thinks he is checking one time per day, then the goal of two or three more blood glucose checks per day will be far less achievable than if Jake were actually already testing one time per day. After establishing a true baseline, setting a goal that is achievable is the next most important aspect of goal setting. Many professionals are inclined to set optimal diabetes self-management as the goal; however, that optimal diabetes self-management is doomed to failure, since most patients cannot achieve such a goal. Finally, a reward should be established for meeting the goal. Since there really are no rewards in diabetes management and people are motivated more by rewards than by the fear of negative consequences, the best way to keep a teen with diabetes motivated to take better care of his or her health is to make sure that there is something in it for him or her. Rewards could include something tangible, such as money, a gift card, a later curfew, or more time with friends.

With regard to goal setting, it is critical that patients be candid about their health behaviors; otherwise, the starting point is not a true baseline from which to measure and establish change. For example, if Jake reports he is checking his blood glucose three times per day but is really checking only once per day, then the goal for more blood glucose checks will be far beyond where Jake is beginning. He is likely to feel overwhelmed by the amount of change that is being asked of him. Teens like Jake struggle to be candid about actual health behaviors for fear of disappointing doctors and of feeling like a failure. Doctors, nurses, and other health care providers are sometimes reluctant to elicit from a patient what he or she is actually doing to manage diabetes. They are reluctant because of the frustration, helplessness, and discomfort they feel when hearing about poor diabetes management. So, they can inadvertently become complicit in the teen's attempt to cover up where he or she is falling short in diabetes management. However, getting a true baseline for diabetes self-management allows for setting realistic goals and for achieving measurable change in health outcomes that are directly linked to better self-care. So besides getting a true baseline, it is important to set goals that are attainable in a relatively short period of time. For Jake, who feels beaten down by his diabetes and is always aware of his poor metabolic control, a small success in something like increasing blood glucose checks or taking more insulin before he eats can shift some of the negative connotations attached to diabetes care.

After the goal is set, it is important to establish a reward tied to the goal completion. Rewards should be things that teens would already do for themselves and that are small but symbolic of a job well done. For example, for adding one more blood glucose check during the course of the day, Jake would earn the reward of getting a movie for the weekend and watching it with friends. Of course, Jake could choose to get the movie and watch it regardless of whether he met the goal. However, the act of revealing his goal to another person, such as a health care provider, will serve as a motivator for him to reward himself only if he meets his goal. In helping teens to craft their goals and rewards carefully, professionals will increase the chances that these patients will be successful. Also, this approach will allow for more positive interactions between health care providers and teens. Going to clinic will be more than just having to be reminded of what isn't going well and what more needs to be done. Instead, it will be an opportunity for both health care providers and teens to enjoy successes.

Giving Jake and his parents the "elephant/rider" analogy allows them to understand that it is normal to struggle with doing the right and rational thing about diabetes care. It allows for seeing Jake not as someone who is unmotivated to take care of his diabetes, but instead as someone who is exhausted by having to make rational decisions all day in many more areas than just diabetes. It allows for problem solving around "feeding the elephant" versus "fighting with the elephant." There has to be a balance; otherwise, the elephant will exert its power and follow its emotion. So feeding the elephant involves some enjoyment, some special treats, something more than just always following the diabetes management plan. Thinking in this way will also allow for clarifying the path for the elephant. It's not enough to simply say, "Jake, you need to take all of your Lantus." The rider needs more direction to get the elephant on the path. Instead, parents and professionals can help Jake identify times when he is likely to miss his Lantus as well as times when he is likely to remember to take it.

5
Parent-Teen Relationships and Diabetes

Most parents make the necessary shifts in parenting to accommodate the changing developmental needs of children as they mature into adolescents. However, some parents struggle with changing their parenting approach to something that is consistent with what adolescents need (Robin 1989).

Parenting Adolescents

Parents provide children with three primary parenting components: involvement, affection, and control. Research has shown that when children are very young, parents are highly involved and affectionate, and exert a great deal of control over their children's lives. That same research demonstrates that as children develop into adolescents, parents become much less involved, show significantly less affection, but continue to exert a great deal of control over their children's lives (Roberts 1984). Developmentally, these changes in parenting are just the opposite of what teens need as they move away from childhood. Instead of less involvement, less affection, and high control, teens need continued involvement from parents, a different type of affection from parents, and significantly less control from parents.

The transition in parenting from childhood to adolescence can be difficult. Parents may wonder how to stay involved with teens, given that teens are often pushing to do more with their friends instead of family. Examples of how parents might stay involved in a teen's life include staying at parties with their teen, supervising their teen's social interactions, knowing the names of their teen's friends, and communicating with the parents of these friends. The shift in type of affection from childhood to adolescence might involve parents transitioning from engaging in a lot of parent-initiated hugging and kissing to sitting close to a teen while watching television. Finally, shifting power and control is something that most parents struggle with during their teen's adolescence. However, slowly shifting power and control to a teen is a necessary and important developmental demand that will result in the teen taking on more responsibility while affording the teen more freedoms. Although there has not been any similar research on parents of youth with diabetes (i.e., longitudinally tracking parenting from childhood to adolescence), Wysocki (1992) has demonstrated that parent-teen relationships are no different for youth with diabetes than they are for youth without diabetes.

The need for a shift in power and control is at least as important for teens with diabetes as it is for their otherwise healthy peers. Teens with diabetes and their parents go through all the developmental challenges that teens without diabetes and their parents go through. In fact, the shift in power and control often happens early for teens with diabetes and their parents because of the demands of diabetes management and the need of the teens to function as independent decision-makers and problem-solvers when away from their parents. In diabetes, this sets up a paradox for teens and their parents, in that teens have power and control over their diabetes and they are expected to take on the responsibility of managing their diabetes independently, yet these same teens are not afforded the same freedom in dealing with non–diabetes-related issues such as curfew, school, and peer relations.

Family Problem Solving

Most parents and teens do not have a structured approach to problem solving, and as a result some parents continue to apply the same top-down approach they successfully used when their children were younger. Because adolescence can be a time of increased conflict between parents and teens, it is imperative for these families to have conflict-resolution skills to avoid mounting family tension. This is particularly important for teens with diabetes and their parents, given the well-established relationship between parent-teen conflict, diabetes self-management, and metabolic control. As conflict increases, diabetes self-management decreases and metabolic control worsens (Harris 2001, Anderson 2004). A structured problem-solving approach that helps families to shift control from parents to teens without undermining parental authority, and that simultaneously reduces conflict, can help families of teens with diabetes. Such an approach allows families to navigate typical diabetes-related problems as well as more general parent-teen problems. (See Figures 5.1 and 5.2 for a problem-solving guide and a problem-solving worksheet.)

Several issues are important to consider when implementing problem solving with families of teens with diabetes. First, do not assume that educated and/or higher socioeconomic status (SES) families need less direction with problem-solving skills than less educated and/or lower SES families. Our clinical experience has demonstrated that regardless of educational level or SES, families with a history of failure at conflict resolution are also likely to struggle with the problem solving around diabetes-related and non–diabetes-related issues.

The second issue to consider when implementing problem solving is that of "problem definition." During the initial explanation of problem solving, the family should be told that parents and teens are not viewed as problems. Instead, the family is told that problems exist between parents and teens. However, when a problem is defined, it is often characterized as one person's problem. For example, when parents and teens argue about blood glucose checking, it is easy to define the problem as "the teen not checking blood glucose enough." Instead, it is better to define the problem as "different views about the number of blood glucose checks necessary for good diabetes control." The second definition construes the problem as existing "between people," thus allowing for the problem to be resolved through compromise, versus a change on only one person's part.

The third issue regarding implementation of problem solving is helping family members to differentiate between "agreeing with" and "understanding" the individual defining the problem during "reflective listening." To get past this hurdle, we recommend telling the family that family members will likely disagree about their problems, and that agreeing about the problems does not make them any more solvable. In addition, helping the family to understand one another's viewpoint reduces debating, decreases conflict (e.g., yelling, interrupting), and facilitates negotiation. Finally, it is essential that all family members have a role in implementing the problem solving at home, so that everyone is contributing to the solution.

FIGURE 5.1. PROBLEM-SOLVING GUIDE

Step 1: Problem Definition (What is the problem?)
a. Select one problem to be discussed.
b. Have one family member state his or her view of the problem in clear terms, using "I-statements" and avoiding accusations (e.g., I feel angry because ...).
c. Discuss this problem only; stay focused; do not bring up the past or other issues.

Step 2: Set Goal (What would you like to happen?)
a. Have family members choose a goal to work on.
b. Have the family discuss the chosen goal.
c. Write down the goal in clear, achievable terms.

**Step 3: Brainstorm Ways to Accomplish the Goal
(How are we going to get it done?)**
a. Ask family members to take turns listing ways to accomplish the goal.
b. Be creative; anything goes. Encourage family members to be silly while they come up with potential solutions, as humor tends to help.
c. Do not judge any of the suggestions made at this time.
d. Write down ALL suggestions; stop after 8–10 ideas are listed.

Step 4: Evaluation (Is this a good idea?)
a. Have each family member rate each solution as positive (+) or negative (–).
b. Try not to rate the idea a certain way based on who came up with it.
c. Choose one of the suggestions with the most pluses to work on first.

Step 5: Action Plan (What is going to happen?)
a. Decide on a length of time before the family reevaluates the goal.
b. Write down a plan for monitoring the progress of the goal.
c. Give each family member a role.

Step 6: Revision of Goal (What happened?)
a. After the trial period, evaluate the success or failure of the goal.
b. If necessary, go back through the steps until the problem is solved.

FIGURE 5.2. PROBLEM-SOLVING WORKSHEET

Problem Definition: _____

Goal: _____

Ways to Accomplish Goal:	Evaluation: (+ or –)		
	P1	P2	Teen
1.			
2.			
3.			
4.			
5.			
6.			
7.			
8.			
9.			
10.			

Parents as a Source of Support

A considerable amount of research demonstrates the positive impact that social support has on health behaviors and health status. Lack of social support has been linked to the onset and progression of health problems; the presence of social support has been linked to recovery. For teens with diabetes, support from parents has been assumed to be a positive influence. However, in some instances, support from parents becomes a destructive force. Based on the writings by Barbara Anderson and James Coyne (1991), the concept of *miscarried helping,* also known as *emotional over-involvement,* outlines how the good intentions of others in supporting an individual with a chronic health condition can result in interpersonal conflict, poorer health behaviors, and poorer health outcomes (see Figure 5.3).

How a situation or event is initially defined usually predicts how it continues to be experienced. If the diagnosis of diabetes is initially defined as a crisis by the family, then family members begin offering aid to the teen and begin pulling together just as they would in any crisis. However, as time goes by after the initial diagnosis of diabetes, it is no longer a crisis, and the demands on the family change. For example, the longer a teen has diabetes, the less emotional involvement by individual family members is warranted. Instead, as the time from diagnosis increases, family members are needed more for validation and instrumental support (e.g., help with ordering diabetes supplies, making doctor appointments). When families fail to change their initial construction of the diagnosis of diabetes, over-involvement and miscarried helping are likely to emerge.

As the teen with diabetes matures, the costs of caregiving become more apparent. Parents of teens with diabetes may experience anxiety, role strain, and general distress as the family begins establishing more routines around diabetes management. The parents may begin to realize that much of their teen's day-to-day care is their teen's responsibility and not under their control. This realization often causes the parents a great deal of anxiety. In addition, the general day-to-day routine becomes more complicated as the daily demands of managing diabetes are superimposed on the family's life. As the burdens of caregiving increase, the positive aspects of the relationship between the teen and his or her family members can become tainted with negativity. In addition, the parents and other family members can evidence significant psychological distress in the face of dealing with a teen with diabetes.

Most individuals are comfortable with receiving care in a crisis. However, once the crisis subsides, it becomes increasingly uncomfortable to receive care from others. The teen may feel some guilt or shame as the relationship with the helper continues to be unbalanced. Consequently, the teen may struggle with self-esteem as this dependency continues and he or she continues to be viewed by others as "impaired." This is even more of an issue as teens become more adept at managing their own health—at a time when teens are trying to develop their own identity separate from their parents.

Example of a Parent-Teen Exchange Gone Awry

Teen comes home from school and just as he or she enters the house, the following exchange occurs:

Parent: Hey, Kari, did you remember your lunchtime shot?

Teen: Yes, Mom!

Parent: Did you check your blood glucose? What was your lunchtime number?

Teen: I don't know. Probably 100-something.

Parent: What do you mean, you don't know? Kari, let me see your meter.

Teen: No!

Parent: If you don't let me see your meter, you're not going out tonight.

Teen: What? Really? That's not fair!

As time goes on, the real and imagined burdens experienced by the family can become emotionally draining and result in family members feeling trapped and resentful. This is even more evident when the teen's health either deteriorates or does not improve despite everyone's help. The problem, once defined as a crisis, is redefined as a burdensome experience that has left family members overwhelmed, drained, and generally unhappy. Soon after diagnosis, many families report that the diagnosis has had positive effects, such as bringing family members together, improving the health behaviors of all family members, or enabling parents and teens to discuss issues that were previously uncomfortable to address or deal with.

Families may initially view diabetes as something that will stabilize with treatment; however, over time, this may shift into an assumption that diabetes is something that may not respond to treatment or is unpredictable in its course. The initial construction of the illness is replaced with a new construction focused on whether the teen is managing his or her diabetes adequately. As more focus is placed on the teen's health behaviors and failures in managing his or her diabetes, the poorer the teen's health behaviors become. This then opens the door to finger-pointing and blame-gaming for poor health outcomes.

With the redefinition of the problem and the reconstruction of diabetes, the family members redouble their efforts to try to help the teen more successfully manage his or her illness, with the health outcomes determining success or failure. This is the point of over-involvement on the helper's part. The helper becomes more and more invested in the outcomes, which now define the helper's success or failure. In addition, the helper begins to view the teen as doing things to undermine both the help and successful diabetes management (Harris 2008).

The *fundamental attribution error* tells us that we are prone to view others' misbehavior as characterological, while understanding our own misbehavior to be situational or context-dependent (Ross 1977). The teen's poor diabetes outcomes are now explained by the parent as a "character trait" evidenced by the teen. The teen senses his or her family member's judgments about why he or she is not doing better, and interpersonal conflict ensues. Rather than focusing on solutions for better diabetes management, the parent and teen focus on each other's character flaws, thus further jeopardizing the child's health. While many psychosocial interventions in diabetes focus on increasing support, there are few if any that deal with the identification and amelioration of the negative impact of parental support on diabetes management.

FIGURE 5.3. MISCARRIED HELPING PARADIGM

Youth has an increase in blood glucose values, experiences poorer metabolic control.

Parents resent burdens of caregiving without successful outcomes; youth feels guilty for not getting better; youth and parents become polarized regarding disease management; unhealthy levels of parent-child conflict emerge.

Parents worry about youth's health and want to help youth with managing and coping with diabetes.

As youth withdraws, parents become more suspicious of youth's health behaviors, start making suggestions about how best to deal with diabetes management.

As the youth's health worsens, parents may accuse and criticize out of frustration; parents begin to question youth about adherence to treatment.

Youth feels blamed and unsupported by parents; youth withdraws from parents.

Case Example

Reid is a 16-year-old male with diabetes. Reid lives with his mother, father, and two younger sisters, aged 9 and 11 years. Reid was diagnosed with diabetes when he was 10 years old. Reid has been on an insulin pump ever since he was diagnosed and is quite independent in taking care of his diabetes. Reid's metabolic control has always been excellent, although his A1C values recently increased slightly from 7.5% to 8.2%. Reid is a competitive athlete and an excellent student. Reid's parents expect a great deal out of Reid and his sisters.

Reid had always been responsive to his parents' requests and had never really shown much defiance. But in the last year, Reid has been challenging his parents more and more and showing more signs of defiance. Reid's parents are extremely worried about his worsening metabolic control and are concerned that he is not as vigilant about his diabetes self-management as before. Reid's escalating defiance has produced a substantial amount of conflict between Reid and his parents. His parents are unaccustomed to his being defiant or challenging their authority, and as a result have resorted to yelling and to using more coercive and controlling methods that were successful when he was younger.

In terms of his diabetes, Reid reports that he continues to manage it as he always has and is perplexed about why his A1C has risen from 7.5% to 8.2%. Reid reports feeling that his parents unfairly accuse him of mismanaging his diabetes and allowing his metabolic control to worsen. Reid's parents feel like Reid is not working as hard on his diabetes care as he should and don't understand why he won't accept their help to get things back on track.

Assessment and Intervention

The changes in parenting needed to more successfully negotiate the parent-child relationship as Reid matures from childhood to adolescence can be understood by thinking of Reid as a dog that is maturing into a cat (Lara 1996, Harris 2006). Dogs are very dependent, always happy to see you, relatively easy to discipline, and very affectionate, and they need you to regulate their food, among other things. Cats are very independent, do not greet you when you arrive home, are difficult to discipline, are affectionate only on their terms, and don't need you to regulate their food. This analogy is a very simple, effective, and memorable way to help parents apply research on development to more successfully shift from parenting a child to parenting an adolescent.

In Reid's case, he needs less and less from his parents; however, faced with his normal health maturation into an adolescent, his parents are struggling to understand the change from his once "dog-like" personality into his more "cat-like" personality. Instead of accommodating this change, Reid's parents appear to be forcing the old strategies of parenting a child onto an adolescent. As a result, Reid is responding as one might expect a cat to respond when treated like a dog. His parents' behavior is akin to putting a leash on a cat and trying to get it to walk around with them.

In addition to the struggles that Reid's parents are having with the need to shift their parenting strategies as Reid matures, they are also struggling with how to best help Reid with his diabetes. Clearly, Reid and his parents are caught in a cycle of miscarried helping. Reid is having some problems with his diabetes management, and as a result his parents are trying to help. Reid's diabetes management is not getting better and so his parents are redoubling their efforts to help him rather than looking more closely at what he actually needs. Reid implicitly feels the pressure from his parents and interprets their over-involvement as mistrust of his ability to care for his diabetes. Likewise, Reid's parents think that he is not trying hard enough, and they begin feeling like he doesn't care about taking care of his diabetes.

The initial phase of treating miscarried helping by parents of teens with diabetes begins with all family members discussing realistic expectations about the teen's diabetes. Myths about diabetes and diabetes care are dispelled. Psychoeducation that includes information on the onset, course, and progression of the teen's diabetes is necessary, as many parents and teens only had the initial education at diagnosis. In addition, discussion is facilitated about diabetes management issues and potential roles for family members in assisting with the teen's diabetes care.

Next, there is a discussion of the family's past and present helping process. This offers family members the opportunity to make explicit their ideas about helping the teen. In addition, the teen has the opportunity to discuss what he or she needs from family members in regard to diabetes management and coping. The family can be provided with direction on how to avoid personalizing the teen's diabetes and how to avoid evaluating their helping based on how well the teen is controlling his or her blood glucose.

Families are then instructed in basic communication skills. Communication-skills training involves identifying disease-specific language as well as the implicit meaning of communication about the teen's diabetes. All family members are educated about psycholinguistics and the impact of language on behavior and psychological functioning. Communication errors are identified along with alternatives for talking about problems.

Finally, the family is guided through a structured problem-solving model. This model focuses on making family members' roles in diabetes management explicit and on coming up with solutions that involve all family members, in order to distribute the burdens of disease management. This offers opportunities for interdependence and the establishment of healthier emotional boundaries between family members. Then the family will be asked to discuss and brainstorm how things will be handled when miscarried helping begins to appear.

6
Mood

A dolescence is full of emotional changes and seemingly rapid swings between the extremes of emotions. The teen with type 1 diabetes is not spared these emotional changes and swings, and, in fact, is at risk for more struggles with emotions. The data are clear on two points: 1) in general, teens are at increased risk for depression and anxiety compared to other age-groups, and 2) teens with type 1 diabetes experience more distress and depression than their peers without diabetes. In this chapter, we will highlight why teens with type 1 diabetes are at increased risk for distress and depression, how distress and depression affect diabetes management, and what is available to clinicians to help teens when they become distressed or depressed.

Definitions

For the purposes of this chapter, *distress* is defined as a collection of psychological symptoms that are uncomfortable, frequent, and disruptive to everyday functioning. Psychological distress may look like depression or anxiety, but is likely not diagnosable as a disorder. Further, distress specific to diabetes can be characterized as *diabetes distress* or *diabetes burnout*. *Depression* is defined as "a common mental disorder that presents with depressed mood, loss of interest or pleasure, feelings of guilt or low self-worth, disturbed sleep or appetite, low energy, and poor concentration." This is the definition adopted by the World Health Organization.

Rates and Consequences

The occurrence of depression and other emotional problems among teens with diabetes is alarmingly higher than in general population samples. Clinically elevated depressive symptoms are present in 15–25% of adolescents with type 1 diabetes. The rates of general psychological distress are even higher. Further, in one of the few longitudinal studies of youth with type 1 diabetes, 50% of teens followed for 10 years after diagnosis met diagnostic criteria for a psychological disorder at some point during those 10 years (Kovacs 1997). This striking percentage is at least twice that of what would be expected in the general population (Lewinsohn 2000). These data suggest that youth with type 1 diabetes, particularly adolescents, are at two to three times the risk for experiencing significant psychological distress and receiving a diagnosis of depression than their peers without diabetes.

By itself, depression is uncomfortable and disrupts social and academic functioning. For the teen with diabetes, depression is also disruptive to diabetes management and control. Depression and distress are associated with less frequent blood glucose monitoring, poorer diabetes management, higher A1C values, and recurrent diabetic ketoacidosis. The reasons for poorer diabetes management by teens who are depressed include difficulties initiating care and sustaining engagement in care, as well as hopelessness that what they do will make a difference in how well they manage diabetes. It is a common misconception that teens just do not want to take care of their diabetes. The more likely scenario is that there are competing emotional demands, priorities, and needs that make it difficult to fully engage in diabetes management.

Identification of Distress and Depression

The first step in helping teens with type 1 diabetes who are experiencing distress, depression, or other problematic psychological functioning is to identify the problem. The U.S. Preventive Services Task Force recommends screening for depression for all youth aged 12–18 years. Given the higher risk for depression in teens with type 1 diabetes, screening in pediatric diabetes clinics is critical. While relatively few data exist on the implementation of such screening programs, it can be done efficiently and successfully. For example, a team at Cincinnati Children's Hospital undertook screening as a quality improvement project. They were able to screen 95% of their teens with type 1 diabetes across a year (n = 562). In the cases of a positive screen for elevated depressive symptoms or suicidal ideation, they provided a more thorough assessment of depression and treatment-planning suggestions (Corathers 2013). This team notes, and it has been noted elsewhere in the literature, that the biggest barrier to systematic psychological screening in pediatric diabetes clinics is a lack of resources to deal with positive screens. With that in mind, below are options for screening for depression in your pediatric clinic that encompass having medical providers do the screening and/or having an experienced mental health professional (social worker, psychologist) conduct the screening and assessment. Note that psychological services can be billed on the same day as medical services.

Screening Questions Used to Open a Clinical Discussion about Depression

At a minimum, consider asking your teenage patients the following questions:

- "During the past month, have you often been bothered by feeling down, depressed, or hopeless?"
- "During the past month, have you often experienced little interest or pleasure in doing things?"

If either question is answered affirmatively, consider follow-up questions about frequency. Further, if the teen is feeling down or has lost interest in activities usually enjoyed on a regular basis (i.e., multiple times weekly), it is important to make a referral to a mental health provider. This can be a social worker, psychologist, counselor, or psychiatrist (although psychiatrists are typically reserved for patients who may require medication management). These questions open a discussion about the teen's emotions. Teens are as scared by these emotions as providers may be about asking about them.

Questionnaires

There are several widely used, validated questionnaires for understanding depression and psychological distress. Although used less often with adolescents, a common tool for adults is the Patient Health Questionnaire (PHQ)-9. This survey is widely used in primary care, and there are recent reports of its appropriate use with teenagers. The PHQ-9 follows diagnostic criteria for depression, and the total score is used to determine the degree of depressive symptoms the respondent endorses in comparison to published norms. The survey can be administered and completed in less than 5 minutes.

For teens, the most widely used questionnaires are the Center for Epidemiologic Studies-Depression (CES-D) scale and the Children's Depression Inventory (CDI). The CES-D contains 20 items; the CDI contains 27 items. Both can be completed in less than 10 minutes. Published norms are available, and in general, scores at or above 16 have been considered elevated on the CES-D, while the CDI cut point has commonly been 13 in the pediatric diabetes literature. Both of these tools get at distress and depression, although they are not used for a diagnosis. If these tools are used, a protocol should be in place to respond to elevated scores. This should involve: *1)* an algorithm for what to do with a certain score (e.g., a score of 5 on the CDI would not require any further action, whereas a score of 16 would require a referral to a social worker or psychologist), *2)* identified individuals who will respond to elevated scores, *3)* a time frame for an appropriate response, and *4)* a follow-up plan for multidisciplinary communication about the identified teen.

Treatment Options

Once a teen's distress or depression has been identified, the next step is to facilitate treatment. This typically occurs via a referral to a mental health professional. While there are just a handful of studies on teens with type 1 diabetes who are also depressed, several other areas of treatment-outcome research align with the diabetes studies to suggest the best treatment options. Before making that referral, it is important to normalize and validate the teen's distress or depression. For example, statements such as "Many teens with type 1 diabetes also feel stressed or depressed," or "Many teens in general feel stressed out," or "It is a lot of work to take care of diabetes and it can sometimes be overwhelming" may be helpful when starting this conversation. It is best to follow these with statements affirming your concern and strong recommendation for psychological treatment, as well as your belief that the teen can feel better and do better. Your sense of hope will give teens a sense of hope that they do not need to suffer.

For teens who receive a diagnosis of major depressive disorder, the best treatment is a combination of antidepressant medication and cognitive-behavioral therapy. This was determined with the Treatment of Adolescent Depression Study and published in the *Journal of the American Medical Association* in 2004 (March 2004). Of note, it appears that cognitive-behavioral therapy was a key ingredient in preventing a relapse of the depression. Keep in mind that these are data on teens with the most severe depression and there are currently no data available for teens with type 1 diabetes and diagnosed depression. It is our collective experience that few parents are interested in having their teens put on another medication (i.e., an antidepressant); thus, the starting point may need to be cognitive-behavioral therapy.

For teens without a diagnosis of depression or for those with elevated levels of psychological distress or depressive symptoms, there are diagnostic options such as *adjustment disorder* and *psychological factors affecting a medical condition*. Such diagnoses should be made by a licensed mental health professional. These teens will likely respond to treatment options such as cognitive-behavioral therapy and problem-solving interventions. The evidence base includes a host of problem-solving interventions that overlap conceptually with cognitive-behavioral therapy. In these interventions, teens are encouraged to identify the problem, brainstorm solutions, select a solution to try, and evaluate the results (and repeat if necessary). This process works well alongside therapeutic strategies to change *distorted thinking* (e.g., "Everything is all my fault" or "Diabetes is horrible and nothing good comes of it") and challenge thoughts that happen automatically in certain situations. At the foundation of any type of therapy, however, is the teen feeling heard, validated, and cared about by the mental health professional. In addition, a professional who is familiar with diabetes and the demands of the daily regimen can often serve a teen and her/his family more effectively than someone without this background.

Case Example

The following case example highlights the recommended steps to take when a teen presents with distress or depression:

Alex is a 15-year-old teen with type 1 diabetes. He was diagnosed 6 years ago and is in the office today for his quarterly diabetes care visit. Even before Alex gets checked in, his mother passes on a recent progress report from school showing that Alex has been slipping academically the past 2–3 months. His usual Bs are now Cs and he's failing one class. Upon reviewing the pump and meter downloads, it is clear that Alex has been checking one to two times daily, the checks are mostly in the 300 range, and he's likely missing boluses, as some days do not show any. All of this is atypical for Alex, as he usually comes in with more frequent checks and an A1C level in the mid-8s.

Today, his A1C value is 9.7%. This, along with the other indicators of problematic management and psychosocial functioning, signals a need to evaluate him for emotional distress. Alex is asked about feeling down, but denies it. He is asked about whether he still likes school and seeing his friends, but he says everything is fine. When asked about his declining grades, he blames the teachers. Because Alex is denying these difficulties, you decide to get him to specifically report on the frequency of doing things he enjoys. He actually cannot remember the last time he went out with his friends other than seeing them at school, and he decided not to play any school sports this term. Upon further inquiry, you find that Alex really does not do much except go to school. And he reports always feeling tired and not sleeping well. With all of these data coming in, it becomes clear that Alex needs to be evaluated by a mental health professional for possible depression. You make a referral to the team's social worker and she helps identify in-network psychologists for your patient.

Some final points to highlight:

1. Although Alex showed signals that he was distressed, any visit with a teen with type 1 diabetes should include the provider posing questions about psychological functioning. Asking questions about or screening for depression should be part of every visit.

2. Try not to blame the teen for poorer management or a rising A1C level. We all know that A1C values are critical parts of the medical management of type 1 diabetes, but they carry such weight in the minds of the people with diabetes and their families that they need to be treated delicately. Further, few teens are motivated to "do better" by knowing that they are not doing well. They have trouble connecting daily management with long-term outcomes.

3. If the treating psychologist does not have experience working with patients with type 1 diabetes, the two of you may need to communicate about diabetes and the nature of diabetes management. Having resources ready for the treating psychologist in the form of websites or handouts will help.

4. If your team does not have a social worker or psychologist on staff, asking for help with referrals from a local community mental health center or partnering with a primary care clinic may provide adequate resources.

7
Technology

Technology has transformed the way type 1 diabetes is managed. Beyond insulin pumps and continuous glucose monitoring (CGM) systems, a host of technologies are aimed at connecting people with diabetes, teaching trends with blood glucose levels in response to dietary intake and physical activity, and facilitating problem solving around diabetes management. The purpose of this chapter is to review those technologies, discuss how and why they work (or don't), and provide recommendations on fitting technology to particular teens. We work from the premise that technologies are not for everyone, but most teens have the ability to use them. Further, we believe that all teens should have access to technologies ultimately aimed at improving their quality of life and health outcomes.

Types of Technologies

There are three types of technologies used in diabetes management: *direct*, *direct+*, and *facilitators*. Technologies in the direct category directly manage diabetes; insulin pumps and blood glucose meters are the most common. The *direct+* technologies are used for direct management but also provide an extra layer of information by showing trends or patterns with management. CGM is the most notable example of a technology in this category, but meter programs that identify trends or patterns are *direct+* as well. Finally, *facilitators* are technologies that were not necessarily developed for diabetes, but that have utility for people with diabetes. Examples include social networking programs to connect people with diabetes, telehealth interventions delivered using Skype, and gaming.

Direct Technologies

The data on insulin pumps are clear: a person with diabetes can achieve improved quality of life and glycemic control while using an insulin pump. Many organizations, including the American Diabetes Association, have practice guidelines for insulin pump use in people with type 1 diabetes (see Phillip [2007] for detailed guidelines). Insurers and state Medicaid offices have been impressed with data on insulin pumps and consider this technology a viable option for caring for type 1 diabetes.

The most recent data from the Type 1 Diabetes Exchange (T1D Exchange), the largest collection of clinical data on pediatric patients with type 1 diabetes, show that of the nearly 25,000 participants in this registry, nearly half are on pumps. Their A1C levels are significantly lower than those of participants on multiple daily injections (Miller 2013). While not every teen may succeed with an insulin pump, we work from the premise that all teens should have access to insulin pumps and, unless contraindicated, should at least try an insulin pump. Fear of technology on the part of the provider or team is not a sufficient reason to refuse access to insulin pumps for patients and families. We recommend conducting a "pump evaluation" before starting pump therapy to be sure teens and their families know what to expect when starting on the pump. Pump evaluation questions could include:

- "What are your reasons for wanting to start pump therapy?"
- "What will be better about being on a pump than doing injections?"
- "What might be worse about being on a pump than doing injections?"
- "Where will you keep the pump on your body?"
- "Do you know others with a pump, and what do they like or dislike about it?"
- "How often will you need to change the pump site?"
- "Is there a sport or activity that you think will be easier with the pump?"

These questions are intended to dispel any myths, such as the pump being a device that allows you to pay less attention to your diabetes. Further, these questions help reveal the advantages and disadvantages for the particular teen. They can assist in weighing if the teen wants more flexibility or if the pump will make it easier to do a certain sport or activity. Body-image concerns about wearing a device may arise from these questions; such concerns should be addressed before the teen starts pump therapy. The teen may also have concerns about losing privacy because the pump is more out in the open for people to see. All of these issues should be addressed before a teen starts pump therapy, and occasional reminders about these topics should be given in ongoing care.

Studies have shown that most teenagers who continue using an insulin pump have improved metabolic control. However, it is important to be aware of the subgroup of teens who miss meal boluses. Teens who miss bolusing for food, versus those who do not miss boluses, also tend to check their blood glucose levels less often and have worse metabolic control: nearly a 1% higher A1C value. They also tend to experience more diabetes-specific distress and perceive their diabetes regimen as more intrusive in their daily lives (Raile 2002, Olinder 2009). Almost 40% of the patients in those studies missed meal boluses during a routine week.

Given the wealth of information on blood glucose meters that is available from companies and product reviews (such as the annual *Diabetes Forecast* review), we will not cover blood glucose meters in this text.

Direct+ *Technologies*

The purpose of *direct+* technologies is to consolidate data in a way that reveals patterns that can then be addressed in daily management. Subsequently, the changes made in response to seeing these trends and patterns should improve overall diabetes control. We would also like to think that *direct+* technologies can also serve as *scaffolding*, particularly for teens. What we mean by *scaffolding* is a temporary framework that provides support and access to more learning. Eventually, successful scaffolding promotes mastery. Scaffolding is a hallmark of education and learning.

The most widely known *direct+* technology is CGM. However, the uptake of CGM in the type 1 diabetes population still rests well below 10% and is probably closer to 5% in pediatric patients. The relatively low uptake is likely due to cost, inconsistent insurance coverage, and the complexity of the technologies for patients and providers alike. While data are still emerging on the efficacy of CGM, it is clear that A1C values can be lowered and severe hypoglycemia reduced or prevented when CGM is used. That is the critical part—*when* it is used. Studies looking at CGM use suggest that you need to use the device for 6 or more days in a row to see an improvement in metabolic control. However, few studies include teens and in those that do, there is generally less uptake of CGM by teens. Thus, more research and clinical evidence are needed to determine the barriers to CGM use in teens, and how to facilitate its uptake.

CGM can be efficacious and serve as scaffolding for a teen in several ways. First, by setting alerts for high and low levels on the CGM device, the teen is learning to respond to early warning signs. Too often teens rely on their own feelings of what their blood glucose levels are, and often they are incorrect when guessing their own values. By having a true alert signaling that they need to pay attention to their diabetes, they are learning to respond to data-driven information instead of just waiting until they "feel" low or high.

Second, CGM technology provides information about the patient's trends. It offers data about where levels have been and where they are going, as well as data about how quickly they are getting there (information about both the direction and the rate of change). These data help teens prevent highs and lows, because they now have information that allows them to predict where their numbers are going. Too often, teens wait until the extremes to do something about their diabetes; they are already too low or too high. By using alarms and examining trends, they can take the appropriate measures to avoid the uncomfortable and possibly unsafe scenario of extreme highs or lows.

Finally, teens can learn what different foods and physical activities do to their blood glucose levels. They may be surprised by how certain foods lead to rapidly changing blood glucose levels, and either alter their eating habits the next time or alter their insulin timing and/or dose. The immediate feedback on food and physical activity allows the teen to incorporate the information into regimen changes, typically with the help of the team. While these skills may not come on board early in the course of CGM use, teens are developing them and will use them later on in adulthood.

Not enough data exist to fully understand the psychological impact of CGM use. However, the few studies on the topic in adults or adolescents suggest that there are no negative consequences of CGM use and that users may experience reduced fear of hypoglycemia. More studies need to be conducted to understand the direct psychological impact of CGM on the user. Of note, several qualitative studies conducted at the Joslin Diabetes Center in adults with type 1 diabetes and their caregivers demonstrate partner benefits as well. Partners take comfort in having an additional monitor of potential hypoglycemia with CGM use, particularly overnight.

Facilitator Technology

The final category includes a host of technologies not typically created for patients with diabetes, but with significant promise for optimizing diabetes management and outcomes. Facilitators engage the teen in a novel way, reduce the burden related to the use of the diabetes technology, and serve as scaffolding for learning. The basis for using these technologies is that the evidence base tells us that simply targeting the change of a behavior (e.g., trying to increase the number of blood glucose checks in a day from two to three) will not be successful if other variables are not considered. Those other variables include perceiving the behavior as important, as time-saving, and as at least moderately fun. The result of using facilitator technologies can be improved problem-solving skills, reduced burden, and more enjoyment doing a necessary activity.

Linking a behavior to a reward within diabetes management can be helpful and can be accomplished with facilitator technologies. For example, several studies have used text messages as reminders to check blood glucose levels as well as to highlight trends, depending on the user's levels. Programs conducted at Vanderbilt University and the Joslin Diabetes Center have demonstrated initial uptake and moderate sustainability over time (Kumar 2004, Mulvaney 2012). They have also demonstrated increased checking frequency and trends toward improvements in A1C values. Text messaging in itself is unlikely to lead to substantial overall improvement in management, but it appears to be a strong hook for engaging teens in their care. Once they are hooked, other interventions that promote problem solving or breaking down barriers can be used.

One of the best-researched areas in this type of technology has been whether effective behavioral interventions that are typically conducted in person can be conducted over the Internet. Two compelling examples come from Coping Skills Training (CST), from the team at Yale University, and from the investigators of Behavioral Family Systems Therapy (BFST) at Oregon Health and Science University, described in more detail in Chapter 8. Both CST and BFST were tested over the Internet (BFST via Skype) and found to be at least as effective as in-person intervention, and potentially more effective. Interestingly, in the BFST Skype study, participants who used Skype were more likely to keep virtual appointments than face-to-face ones, and they ended up with more total visits than the face-to-face participants (Harris 2012a). Facilitating health behavior change and positive outcomes via a well-known and accepted technology serves to increase reach to the patient population and is in a "language" that many teens can understand.

Another facilitator technology involves gaming. Gaming is a staple of many teens' lives, whether played on a TV, computer, or mobile device. To hook teens, games have to be innovative, visually appealing, and based in a system that reinforces and rewards strong play. For example, contingencies are powerful reinforcers in games, as an outcome is directly linked to performing some behavior. In other words, the gamer does X and gets Y. Token economies are also embedded in gaming, meaning that gamers have to perform certain behaviors or complete tasks to increase the size of their "banks." As the bank balance increases, more options are available for spending what has been earned. While data are sparse in youth with diabetes, there are emerging data on adults with diabetes and gaming.

Finally, a popular facilitator is social networking around diabetes. Social networking can happen on websites, via links provided in apps for smartphones, and within online pediatric diabetes communities. However, teens with type 1 diabetes tend not to be high users of these online or mobile resources. While anecdotal, the reasons for this likely include little interest in connecting about diabetes online. Instead, they would rather connect with friends, and if diabetes comes up, that is fine. This scenario is strikingly different from adults with diabetes, who have large online communities and seek support through websites such as TuDiabetes (www.tudiabetes.org) and via bloggers (see *six until me* for an example [www.sixuntilme.com]). Thus, when you attempt to engage teens with type 1 diabetes via social networking, you will likely need to find ways to embed these resources and programs within their existing social networking frameworks.

Case Example

It has been a struggle to find ways to hook 14-year-old Marta into taking care of her diabetes. She was diagnosed just over a year ago and was engaged in care for the first 9 months. For the past few months, she has not wanted to check as frequently and has not shifted her relatively predictable schedule of insulin administration to adjust for wide-ranging blood glucose levels and higher numbers. Marta is struggling with what seems like a second diagnosis, where she has to ramp up the frequency and intensity of diabetes care because she needs more insulin and has wider-ranging blood glucose levels.

Marta voiced interest in the pump early on, but now is more skeptical. Her understanding of the pump is that it basically just does the same thing as injections and there are not many advantages to its use. She heard this from a teen in her ninth-grade class who refuses to use the pump. Upon hearing this, Marta's diabetes care team has an opportunity to provide more education about the pump and its potential advantages over insulin injections. Instead of doing the standard education, which was provided early on in the course of her diabetes care, the team decides to bring in several young adults who have been successfully using the pump. They are all former patients of the practice and can give Marta some examples of the ways the pump has helped them better manage diabetes. Further, they all have different pumps, including some with colorful or self-designed skins that are more visually appealing. Marta's interest is piqued and she follows through on getting the pump started.

Imagine Marta several years later, after she has just completed her first year of college classes. She decided to stay home and take classes at a local community college while she works. This made her feel a little more secure in caring for her diabetes, and also alleviated her parents' concerns about her being far away from home. However, Marta is feeling a little trapped by the constant blood glucose checks and by her parents' nagging. Marta discusses an interest in something that will help her feel a little more autonomous, although she is not sure what that is. The team discusses CGM with her as well as options for trend programs associated with apps that she could use with her smartphone. She decides to try GlucoseBuddy online, and after several weeks, feels it was helpful. However, she notices that it is not helping as much with preventing lows, which she has frequently, given her tight schedule between work and school. In other words, she needs a real-time alert for herself. The team works with Marta to start CGM and gives her about a month of trials before she feels comfortable with the system. Because Marta needed to "switch things up" to stay engaged in her own diabetes care, she benefited from trying several different technologies.

8
Repeat DKAs

I t is well known that adolescence is the most difficult time to control blood glucose levels, and despite the fact that most teens with diabetes weather this period in their lives without excessive hospitalizations for DKA, a subgroup of teens evidence a major deterioration in their metabolic control and are repeatedly hospitalized for DKA. Typically these teens maintain double-digit A1C values. They are often referred to as "frequent fliers" or "train wrecks" by members of their diabetes treatment team. Such teens are often difficult to treat, resulting in increased time commitments and stress for their health care providers. Furthermore, because of the chronic and difficult-to-treat nature of diabetes, substantial costs are associated with the management of young people with diabetes.

What is known about this subgroup of teens and their families is that they are buried under a mound of life stressors and challenges that make it difficult to properly attend to diabetes care. For example, in a sample of 20 teens with diabetes who were hospitalized repeatedly for DKA (three times in the past 6 months), a disproportionate number lived in single-parent families and 63% of the teens' parents were either unemployed or underemployed (Harris 2013a). Moreover, the teens and their parents suffered from psychosocial, behavioral, and mental health problems at a much higher rate than did families of teens with diabetes not repeatedly hospitalized for DKAs (Harris 2013a).

Many of the hospital admissions for DKA are avoidable. In this subgroup of repeatedly admitted teens, DKA episodes are rarely due to illness or other uncontrollable factors. Instead, the teens' psychosocial circumstances contribute to poor adherence, poor access to care, and poor metabolic outcomes. Intensive behavioral health interventions that address teens with poorly controlled diabetes have proven effective in improving adherence to treatment, improving overall psychosocial functioning, and reducing avoidable hospitalizations (e.g., Harris 2003, Wysocki 2007, Ellis 2008a, Harris 2013a). However, many youth do not have access to integrated care with behavioral health professionals who specialize in the care and treatment of youth with complex medical conditions. Either because families live too far from tertiary medical centers that provide specialized care to youth with diabetes or because youth are underinsured, getting the necessary specialized care is often difficult, placing these youth at high risk for deteriorating health and repeated hospitalizations due to suboptimal adherence.

Besides being a symptom of our poorly organized health care system and causing significant problems for health care providers, patients, and their families, the lack of multidisciplinary integrated care for youth with diabetes creates a huge financial burden on both the health care system and the insurers (Harris 2013a).

With adherence rates for most complex medical conditions hovering around 50%, but plummeting as low as 10% for certain health behaviors (DiMatteo 2002), nonadherence costs the U.S. alone as much as $100 billion annually (Osterberg 2005). It is also estimated that upwards of 50% of hospitalizations for children with complex medical conditions are due to poor adherence to treatment. While the mean cost of the hospitalization of a child is approximately $5,200 (Yu 2011), the cost of the hospitalization of a child with a complex medical condition is considerably more. For example, the mean cost of one hospitalization for DKA for someone with type 1 diabetes is approximately $15,000 (Kitabchi 2009). Given that many hospitalizations for teens with diabetes are avoidable and likely linked to poor adherence, the cost savings in preventing these hospitalizations can be impressive when one compares the cost of intensive behavioral health care to the cost of repeated hospitalizations linked to poor adherence (Harris 2003, Ellis 2008a, Harris 2013a).

An intervention that specifically targets those youth with diabetes who are repeatedly hospitalized for DKA and whose hospitalizations are avoidable must involve some traditional family-based psychosocial intervention, but these youth also need a substantial amount of care coordination and case management. And although it is important for those working with these youth to have specific diabetes knowledge, they also need to understand the context in which these youth live; otherwise, any intervention implemented has a great likelihood of failing, owing to the many obstacles faced by these youth and their families.

Case Example: Intervention for Repeat DKAs

Recently, an intervention has been developed, implemented, and evaluated for teens who are repeatedly hospitalized for DKA. Below is a diagram (Figure 8.1) of the intervention, known as NICH or Novel Interventions in Children's Healthcare (Harris 2013b). This intervention is grounded in the social ecology of the youth's life, addressing the many contextual factors that can affect adherence to the diabetes treatment regimen and that are often responsible for deterioration in a young person's metabolic control.

As you can see from Figure 8.1, there is simultaneous focus on devel-

FIGURE 8.1. NOVEL INTERVENTIONS IN CHILDREN'S HEALTHCARE (NICH)

CARE COORDINATION
Attend Clinic Appointments
Ensure Transportation to Clinic
Adequate Medical Supplies
Liaison Between Medical Team and Family
Contact Prior to Hospitalization
Care Ambassador/Navigator

BEHAVIORAL FAMILY SYSTEMS THERAPY
Family-Based Problem Solving
Communication Skills Training
Family Roles and Structure
Management of Family Conflict
Establish Proper Supervision

CASE MANAGEMENT
Working with School
Assistance with Job/Work
Interface with DHS
Access to Drug/Etoh Treatment
Assistance with DV Issues
Insecure Housing
Other Resources for the Family

© 2012 Michael A. Harris, PhD. DHS, Child Protective Services; DV, domestic violence.

oping specific problem-solving skills with a family of a child with diabetes, while also serving as a Novel Interventions in Children's Healthcare (NICH) liaison between the family and the diabetes team and functioning as a case manager in addressing the many contextual obstacles that are indirectly related to diabetes management.

Although the success of innovative programs like NICH is largely a function of the people involved, some distinct and necessary attributes of NICH are reproducible. Most importantly, the intervention must be grounded both theoretically and empirically. The theoretical base of NICH guides the interventionist in implementation of the empirically supported interventions with purpose and direction that best address the needs of the families by bridging what is proven to be effective with real-world challenges and the multitude of demands of life. NICH is grounded in Urie Bronfrenbrenner's (1979) social-ecological theory of human development. Attending to the normal developmental demands of youth with complex medical conditions is critical, along with analyzing and understanding the impact of the various systems or contexts in which these youth live.

Bronfrenbrenner's theory attends to a child's development within the context of the systems that impact the child both directly and indirectly. Bronfrenbrenner describes five distinct systems: microsystems, meso-systems, exosystems, macrosystems, and chronosystems. Microsys-tems encompass a child's immediate surroundings and environment (e.g., family, school, peers, health care system). Mesosystems are the linkages between a child's microsystems (e.g., interactions between parents and health care providers). Exosystems are those systems that a child is not directly involved in, but that have the potential to affect him or her, such as a parent's work schedule, local and county organizations, and health insur-ance. Macrosystems represent cultural values, customs, and laws. Finally, chronosystems refer to the timing of developmental and life events that a child may react differently to depending on his or her age and develop-ment (e.g., being diagnosed with type 1 diabetes as a child rather than as an adolescent).

Without a fundamental theoretical paradigm, a program like NICH is merely a set of evidence-based interventions that cannot be successfully implemented outside controlled conditions and in the unpredictable world of real-life challenges. As a result, NICH cases are conceptualized based on development within the context of systems that have both direct and indirect impact on the child.

Although grounded in Bronfrenbrenner's social-ecological theory of human development, the specific interventions used in NICH are drawn largely from Behavioral Family Systems Therapy (BFST) (Robin 1989). BFST has received notable attention and is one of the most researched behavioral health interventions for youth with chronic health conditions. BFST is a structured, manualized intervention with four primary components: problem-solving training, communication-skills training, cognitive restructuring, and family-systems interventions (Wysocki 2001).

Problem-solving training entails teaching family members specific skills for recognizing issues causing interpersonal or other conflicts and a process for successfully generating and testing solutions for those issues in a collaborative manner. Communication-skills training emphasizes language and phrasing that can be used during family exchanges to promote healthy discussions among family members and to avoid blaming or overreacting. Cognitive restructuring involves teaching individuals how to recognize faulty or maladaptive beliefs that may influence actions (e.g., "My son is just lazy. He would take care of his health if he really cared"), as well as strategies for altering those beliefs. Finally, family-systems interventions include approaches that help ensure that appropriate relationship boundaries and relational structures exist within the family (e.g., ensuring parents work together, engendering appropriate negotiation of roles and responsibilities). In combination, the various components of BFST directly target many of the family-functioning and personal variables shown to have an impact on the health status of adolescents with diabetes. Extant literature on BFST highly supports both its efficacy and its effectiveness for adolescents with type 1 diabetes (Wysocki 1997, Wysocki 1999, Wysocki 2000, Wysocki 2001, Wysocki 2006, Harris 2003).

NICH has been successfully implemented with a very diverse population of youth with type 1 diabetes (Harris 2013a). Although NICH interventionists need to have diabetes knowledge to properly address the health behaviors of these youth, they also use a template of interventions to attempt to improve health behaviors and ultimately improve health outcomes.

First, NICH interventionists have sought to establish a strong understanding of the context in which these youth live, including the identification of key players in a child's life who can support the treatment regimen. Second, NICH interventionists have placed great importance on clarifying for the youth and family what health care behaviors are necessary and on providing direction on how to remediate poor health behaviors. Thus, identifying short- and long-term medical goals as well as problem solving around how to reach these goals appeared to reduce barriers to treatment progress. Oftentimes, these young people get discouraged when they are pushed for optimal adherence. Unfortunately, such adherence is often unattainable, given the many challenges they have in their lives coupled with their current baseline of health behaviors being so far from optimal. The short-term goals allow for immediate success and a sense of accomplishment and self-efficacy. The longer-term goals keep optimal adherence as something that is always considered. Third, NICH interventionists emphasize building small health care wins that are attainable and immediate. This concept is exemplified by working toward a goal of checking blood glucose levels one more time per day, as opposed to a goal of perfect adherence. These small wins allow for a shift away from a completely negative experience around one's health and address the need for establishing control over something that feels uncontrollable. Finally, and possibly most importantly, the NICH interventionist serves as the "care ambassador" for the youth and the family, as many of these youth have been marginalized by the health care system and need assistance reengaging in care. The interventionists work to better inform the diabetes care providers of the socioeconomic difficulties and other barriers that young people and their families face on a daily basis, with the intention of increasing medical providers' feelings of empathy and motivation to help them succeed.

Case Example of NICH

Allyson is a 14-year-old female with type 1 diabetes. She lives with her mother and her stepfather. Allyson has struggled to manage her disease since her diagnosis several years ago. She has several other medical conditions, including chronic pain, gastrointestinal issues, and chronic depression/anxiety, which greatly complicate management of her disease. She was kicked out of school because of poor health, which severed one of her only sources of social contact and happiness. Allyson's mother and stepfather are both living with and managing their own conditions and disabilities and doing so without health insurance. Her mother has kidney issues and prediabetes; her stepfather has type 2 diabetes and severe back pain from a work injury. Allyson's maternal grandmother lives with the family and is going through chemotherapy to treat her cancer. The family is under constant threat of eviction, is struggling to find enough food, is unable to pay utilities, and lives more than 150 miles from a major medical center.

Assessment and Intervention

The role of the NICH interventionist is to address those factors in Allyson's life that prevent her from properly managing her diabetes and getting appropriate supervision and support for her diabetes. Often in cases like this, the obstacles to proper diabetes management lie in those aspects of a young person's life that are not directly related to diabetes. In this case, NICH provided school support and succeeded in setting Allyson up in an alternative school program where she can work on mainstreaming back to high school as soon as she is healthy. NICH reengaged the family with local health care providers by contacting the doctors first and giving them the family's back story so that the same mistakes that alienated the doctors from the family in the first place would not recur. NICH got Allyson engaged with a gastroenterologist and an endocrinologist at the local hospital, set up transport to get the family there, supported a move to more suitable housing, and taught/supported/reinforced disease management in the home setting to build the confidence and self-efficacy of the teen and her family. NICH supported Allyson in getting a job and volunteer work outside the home so that she has social contact with peers and feels like she is productive and contributing. NICH supported Allyson and her family in developing the skills to maintain and persevere on their own. The patterns that families like Allyson's develop now, whether positive or negative, will be entrenched for life. Negative patterns lead to a quality of life replete with pain and suffering and come with great cost to the individual and society alike. NICH supports the development of healthy patterns that will produce lasting and positive change.

9
High-Risk Behaviors

Given the dynamic and unfinished nature of cognitive, emotional, and physical development that defines adolescence, many behaviors can be considered high-risk. However, for the purposes of this chapter, we define high-risk as those behaviors that carry with them the potential for serious and harmful consequences. In this chapter, we will cover the high-risk behaviors of sexual activity, substance use, disordered eating, and driving.

Our Assumptions

We work from the premise that the most effective ways to address these high-risk behaviors are prevention and early intervention, followed by more intensive intervention when circumstances dictate. Prevention and early intervention efforts include education, problem-solving skill development, and ongoing monitoring. It might be helpful if each provider and practice develops a plan, created by the members of the clinical team, focusing on prevention efforts for these high-risk behaviors. Specific recommendations for addressing these behaviors follow within each topic discussed.

Another assumption we make is that every child should receive information at an early age, although how much information is given will vary. It is our opinion that these topics should be introduced during the age range of 12–13 years. Data from the Centers for Disease Control and Prevention (CDC) and other studies suggest that youth are being introduced to substances and have opportunities for sexual activity in the middle school years. CDC data show that over 60% of ninth graders have tried alcohol at some point in their lives and over 20% self-identified as sexually active. If you start talking about sex and alcohol at age 14 or 15 years, you will likely miss your chance at prevention.

A final assumption is that the discussion of these topics is non-negotiable; however, who does the discussing is negotiable. Within a multidisciplinary team of physicians, nurses, diabetes educators, psychologists, and social workers, some may be better at discussing certain topics than others. Further, a certain provider may feel uncomfortable discussing a certain topic, in which case that topic will be better addressed by another member of the team. The point is that the information needs to be transmitted, but any of the qualified team members can deliver it.

Sexual Activity

The American Diabetes Association's Standards of Medical Care (American Diabetes Association 2009) recommend preconception counseling starting at puberty. The Standards focus more on females than males, and multiple reports have demonstrated that a program called READY-Girls (Charron-Prochownik 2008, Fischl 2010), developed by Charron-Prochownik and colleagues, is effective. The program has also been shown to be cost-effective, in that it offsets costs associated with unwanted pregnancies. The program works because it increases knowledge and the perceived benefits of reproductive health. Participating girls are more likely to openly discuss sexual topics and engage in safe sexual activity. READY-Girls and other such programs are characterized by a multimedia approach to education and engagement in discussion about reproductive health. Discussions of decision making about sexual activity, safe sex, and planning for pregnancy (at a later date) with type 1 diabetes are critical for general and diabetes health for these young women. It is important to remember that talking about sexual activity does not mean you are encouraging your patients to engage in such activity. However, raising the topic not only increases the likelihood that patients will have the necessary knowledge to make informed decisions, but also lets your patients know that you are a caring adult whom they can turn to for advice and support. Finally, talking with girls about the impact of sexual activity (as with any activity) on blood glucose levels is helpful.

Programs for boys are less common, and most practitioners rely on standard sex education for males with type 1 diabetes. Our opinion is that it is also helpful to discuss specifics about type 1 diabetes. For example, it may be helpful to discuss other activities that are physical in nature (e.g., sports, workouts) to help instruct your teenage male patients with type 1 diabetes about whether adjustments will be needed for insulin dosing during sexual activity. Further, it will be important to discuss how excitement and adrenaline affect blood glucose levels in the particular patient in front of you. Talking with teenage boys about "performance" from a physical standpoint can help them avoid embarrassing situations arising from high or low blood glucose levels. In fact, sometimes the desire for performance is THE motivation for increasing blood glucose checks and missing fewer boluses.

Finally, two other clinical topics are good to assess and discuss, whether you are meeting with a teenage girl or boy. First, discuss how to handle disconnections from the pump (if the teen is on a pump) and when to check blood glucose levels around sexual activity. Second, consider sexual orientation when having discussions related to sexual activity. By phrasing questions about romantic relationships and dating in a gender-neutral way, you create a safer environment for open discussion about sexual activity. For example, instead of asking a 15-year-old boy, "Do you have a girlfriend?" it is better to ask "Are you dating anyone?" And when asking about sexual activity, it is good to ask, "Do you engage in any sort of sexual activity with someone else?" Following up with questions about orientation ("Some people prefer dating boys and some prefer dating girls. Others aren't sure who they prefer. Do you have a preference yet?") and type of sexual activity ("Some people are comfortable cuddling and kissing. Others feel they are ready for more and touch each other naked. Some feel they are ready for intercourse. Where are you in your readiness for sexual activity?") is appropriate and will dictate which topics are discussed next.

Substance Use

Most teens engage in substance use. It is not clear if teens with type 1 diabetes engage in more or less substance use than their peers without diabetes, as study results on this topic are mixed. It is safe to assume that teens with type 1 diabetes are exposed to the same peer pressures and opportunities for substance use as any other teen. However, the potential for negative consequences associated with substance use for teens with type 1 diabetes is substantially higher. Thus, we identify three themes that should be covered when discussing substance use with teens with type 1 diabetes.

First, it is important to tell teens with type 1 diabetes that using substances is more risky because they have diabetes. There is just no way around this fact. Explaining this can lead to a discussion about the importance of being more prepared than others if the decision is made to use substances. Teens should be informed of the direct and indirect effects of substances on blood glucose levels. For example, it would be helpful to have a discussion about how alcohol can increase risk for hypoglycemia by creating an imbalance of sugar and insulin in the system because of the liver's "inability" to produce sugar and clear out alcohol at the same time. Teens seem to respond well to thinking of the liver as "not so smart" and that they have to plan ahead for when the liver is not able to do its primary job (making sugar). Teens forget that nicotine is a substance, but there are clear, direct effects on blood glucose levels from the drug, which also constricts blood vessels and exponentially increases the risk for cardiovascular disease. Sadly, data suggest that more than 17% of youth with type 1 diabetes between the ages of 15 and 19 years smoke, and more than 30% of youth with type 1 diabetes over 20 years of age smoke (Reynolds 2011). Clearly, it is vital that providers counsel teens on avoiding nicotine and cigarette smoking. In fact, fewer than half of teens with type 1 diabetes who smoke report ever being counseled AGAINST smoking—either by their parents or by their diabetes providers (Regber 2007, Reynolds 2011).

We have little data on the direct effect on blood glucose levels of marijuana, ecstasy, amphetamines, and the many other illegal substances. However, all will certainly have indirect effects. For example, marijuana will not likely raise or lower blood glucose levels while being used, but the subsequent "munchies" combined with impaired judgment can lead to forgetting to check blood glucose, missing insulin, and/or miscalculating insulin doses. In sum, an important message for teens to hear is that every substance will have either a direct or an indirect effect on blood glucose levels. Recent data suggest that among youth with type 1 diabetes, 16% of all deaths were related to drug misuse, and 71% of those deaths occurred among youth between the ages of 20 and 29 years (Feltbower 2008). Therefore, we strongly recommend urine toxicology screens for all adolescents admitted to a hospital for high blood glucose levels or for DKA.

A second theme is providing a guide for making informed decisions about substance use. Adolescence is marked by constant concerns about whether one fits in and is liked by peers, and what other teens think. This is fertile ground for succumbing to peer pressure in order to be received more favorably by peers, or not to seem different. A helpful guide for teens with type 1 diabetes, and teens in general, is to make decisions about substance use before being asked. Ask them to consider several different scenarios and encourage them to think through how they would respond if presented with substances (for example, at a school gathering, at a friend's house, and at other places). It will help them when the actual situations happen. Encourage them to come up with actual phrases and plan for how to respond to increased pressure after an initial no. Also, encourage the teen to use diabetes as an out if need be. They may want to say something like, "Yeah, I'd really like to try it, but I really can't because of my diabetes." Some teens may find this explanation to be a good excuse to avoid more peer pressure. The simple "just say no" will not work, so help the teen be as prepared as possible by role-playing and having ready answers.

A third theme is preparation for substance use. Encourage the teen to do three things: 1) have a full stomach before using substances, 2) have a close friend along who is not using substances and who knows the teen has type 1 diabetes, and 3) be very careful and cautious. The first two are relatively straightforward and speak to safety. Teens with type 1 diabetes must have a sober friend with them who knows what to do if problems arise because of diabetes. This can be a bit tricky, as teens need to really think about who the ideal friend will be. Figuring out who will stick by them (even if the cutest person is flirting with them at the party) and how to avoid straining the friendship must all be considered. The "be very careful" plan deals with checking and insulin administration. Teens will ask about what they are supposed to do with their basal (or background) insulin rates while consuming alcohol, for example. They can be generally encouraged to be very careful by cutting back on basal rates and/or not giving full boluses, but they will want to know by exactly how much. In general, teens who are more cautious and conservative with insulin dosing while drinking alcohol have a better chance of not going low later. Of course, it is also important for clinicians to remind their patients that drinking and driving never mix.

Disordered Eating

Teenagers are rarely satisfied with the way they look. Some think they're too short, others too tall. Some think they have bad skin. Some think they have funny-looking noses. Many believe they are overweight. Approximately 11% of all high school students have gone without eating for a full 24 hours in an attempt to lose weight (Centers for Disease Control and Prevention 2010). Eighty percent (yes, 80) of 18-year-old females want to lose weight (Jones 2001). For teenagers who also have diabetes, weight concerns lead to even bigger challenges.

There are many reasons that youth with type 1 diabetes focus on, and struggle with, weight. For example, many youth lose quite a bit of weight before diagnosis. If that diagnosis occurred during the adolescent years, the teenagers probably heard friends telling them that they looked great as they got thinner. In addition, soon after diagnosis, patients often gain back the weight that they lost. This can easily lead to the belief that "insulin makes me fat" (as opposed to understanding that the weight loss was a result of starvation from lack of insulin, and that the weight gain is a sign of health—that taking insulin is allowing their bodies to build back the muscle mass they lost).

Another reason that weight is a challenge for teens with diabetes is the role of puberty. Puberty is a state of insulin insensitivity, which means that most teens are taking more insulin during puberty than they needed to before they began puberty. Sometimes that higher dose of insulin is not decreased when puberty ends, leading teens to eat much more food than they need (to cover the insulin), which in turn leads to inadvertent weight gain.

Researchers who have focused on eating behaviors among individuals with type 1 diabetes have found that disturbed eating behaviors are more common in girls and women with type 1 diabetes than among their healthier peers. Some studies suggest that the prevalence rate may be as high as 25% (Jones 2000, Peveler 2005). Some predictors of disturbed eating behavior include higher BMI (Colton 2007, Olmsted 2008, Markowitz 2009), lower self-esteem (Colton 2007, Olmstead 2008), overt concerns about weight and shape (Olmstead 2008), and depressive symptoms (Olmstead 2008). Sadly, disturbed eating behaviors may be normative, as one study showed that almost half of females between 14 and 18 years of age acknowledged disturbed eating behaviors, such as insulin omission for weight control (Colton 2007).

The medical consequences of disturbed eating behaviors underscore the need for prevention, assessment, and treatment. In one landmark study of 91 adolescents by Rydall (1997), the A1C of those who engaged in disturbed eating behaviors was 11.1%, while the A1C of those without such eating issues was 8.7%. Moreover, when this cohort of individuals was assessed 4 years later, 86% of those who engaged in disordered eating behaviors had evidence of retinopathy, while 24% of those without such disordered behaviors showed signs of this complication. A more recent landmark study by Goebel-Fabbri and colleagues (2008) followed a cohort of 234 women. Participants were asked if they had ever omitted insulin at least once with the goal of losing weight. When those women were assessed 11 years later, those who admitted omitting insulin as a means of weight loss had a mortality rate three times higher than those who did not manipulate insulin to lose weight.

Given the high prevalence of disturbed eating behaviors, and the devastating consequences of such behaviors, it is incumbent upon clinicians to assess their adolescent patients for such potentially dangerous behaviors. What kinds of statements might you hear in the clinic that would suggest your patient is struggling with disturbed eating behaviors? Some patients will make statements such as: "I have to eat too much because of my diabetes," or "I can't lose weight no matter how hard I try," or "Diabetes makes me fat." Similarly, if parents complain that their child is no longer willing to take insulin in front of them, or if a parent reports noticing that the child has recently lost a lot of weight, then the possibility of eating issues should be further addressed. Clinically, you might see elevated A1C values that are moving into the double-digit range. You might notice a marked weight loss in your patient. You might hear unrealistic weight goals. You might learn that your patient has significantly increased physical activity. Finally, you might see an increase in emergency department visits or inpatient admissions due to high blood glucose levels or DKA.

Often, the easiest way to assess for disturbed eating behaviors is simply to ask: "How often do you skip or take less insulin to avoid gaining weight or to lose weight?" If eating issues are not part of the picture, adolescents will state that they never do this. If eating issues are part of the picture, you will hear some interesting stories.

Case Example

Mary, a smart, popular junior in high school, was trying to lose weight but found it nearly impossible. So she decided to disconnect from her pump while she was in school because her mother wouldn't see it there. She kept the pump running in her backpack and wrapped gauze around the pump to absorb the basal insulin as it was being dispensed. She put her pump back on when she got on the school bus to go home and gave herself a bolus of insulin so that when she checked at home, her number wouldn't be "too high." She would do the same thing at night, while she was sleeping. Sometimes she'd use the control solution to show a "good" number on her meter to her mother, and sometimes she'd convince a friend to let her poke the friend's finger to get a "good reading." Mary lost approximately 15 pounds in 2 weeks, but also wound up in the pediatric intensive care unit in DKA.

How can disturbed eating behaviors and insulin omission be prevented? One way is to provide realistic goals for blood glucose averages and ranges during puberty. The goal of perfection sets patients up for a sense of failure. In addition, it is important to openly discuss the issue of possible weight gain after diagnosis and during puberty. Also discuss strategies to minimize weight gain, if that is a safe and healthy goal.

Once you believe that your patient is struggling with disturbed eating behaviors, it is important to have parents take on responsibility for administering all insulin and performing all blood glucose checks. It is also important to realize that your patient has probably been underinsulinized for some time, so ramping up to the amount of insulin actually needed will probably have to be done slowly. Rapid increases in insulin doses cause rapid weight gain, which will not be acceptable for your patients who have been using insulin omissions as a means of weight loss. Therefore, small increases in insulin dosing are recommended. Finally, it is vital that such patients engage in psychological services. Some require inpatient admission, others need a day-treatment program, and some can manage on an outpatient basis. Working with a social worker or psychologist who can assess your patient and recommend treatment options is important.

Driving

Teenage drivers are not safe drivers. They get distracted, cause accidents, and, at times, put others' lives at risk. Teens with type 1 diabetes are no more prone to distraction than other teens, but the additional risk of going low (or high) puts them in a higher-risk category. Data suggest that drivers with type 1 diabetes have more than twice the risk of collisions than do those without diabetes. Even mild hypoglycemia impairs cognitive-motor functioning (important driving skills) and it impairs a person's judgment (another important driving skill) (Cox 2000, Cox 2003, Cox 2009, Cox 2010). Thus, it is important that teens who are planning to drive, or are already driving, be reminded of several requirements.

First, checking blood glucose (or inspecting the CGM display) is what provides access to the keys to the car. No teen should even put a key into an ignition without first checking. Teens need to know both their current blood glucose level and the direction in which they may be heading. It is important to set a range for acceptable driving conditions. This range may be 80–180 mg/dL or some other agreed-upon range. In particular, the upper range may be more flexible, since the majority of diabetes-related driving mishaps are the result of hypoglycemia, not hyperglycemia, as the research of Cox and colleagues at the University of Virginia points out.

Second, the car should be stocked with plenty of accessible treatments for low blood glucose. Such treatments include juices, glucose tablets, and candy. The teen may need to treat a low before the low can be confirmed with a blood glucose check. If teen drivers feel low at any point, they should pull over as soon as possible and check.

Third, any time there are long distances driven, a plan should be in place for routine checking of blood sugars. It may be that every 2 hours is the decided-upon frequency given the journey, but plans for lows and treatment of lows obviously supersede any scheduled checks.

If providers are interested in using driving as a carrot for improving diabetes management control, this approach can sometimes work. It can also backfire (pun intended). If providers want to set clear expectations for getting a driver's license—check before driving in addition to checking X number of times throughout the day—that seems reasonable as long as it is an achievable goal. In other words, a teen checking once a day will not be able to do four to five checks a day immediately.

If teens are encouraged to bring down their high A1C levels so they can drive, reasonable goals should be set that focus on behaviors, not the A1C level. For example, if a teen checking twice daily is routinely running in the 10–11% range for A1C and the team and parents are interested in having that come down, it would make sense to set up a system where specific changes in self-care behaviors are made so that driving is the reward (if the teen wants to drive). For example, this teen could be encouraged to check three times daily (up from two) and make sure all Lantus doses are received during the week (let's say that he is currently missing one to two per week). A system where a parent supervises the Lantus injection and provides positive feedback when it is done can also be part of the plan. If the behaviors are completed, driving can be the reward—even if the teen's A1C level has not come down yet.

10
Transition

The need for planned transition from pediatric to adult health services for youth with chronic illness has been recognized by important stakeholders in health care and in important policy papers on health care, including Healthy People 2010, the Society for Adolescent Medicine, the Royal College of Paediatrics and Child Health, and the consensus statement from the American Academy of Pediatrics, the American Academy of Family Physicians, and the American College of Physicians (American Academy of Pediatrics 2011). Likewise, in a position statement by the American Diabetes Association (Peters 2011), similar recommendations are outlined for transition of the emerging adult with type 1 diabetes. This chapter provides a developmental context for these recommendations and details a four-step transition plan that can be implemented in your clinic.

Emerging Adulthood

Transitioning from pediatric to adult care typically occurs in late adolescence and early adulthood, a time of vulnerability often characterized by poor judgment and decision-making, risk-taking behaviors, and emotional reactivity. Arnett coined the term *emerging adulthood* for the period between 18 and 25 years of age, recognizing that maturation is still occurring and many milestones still need to be achieved. In a seminal study, Arnett (2000) asked individuals between the ages of 18 and 24 years what attributes make someone an adult. Four specific achievements were cited: *1)* the ability to accept responsibility for oneself, *2)* the ability to make independent decisions, *3)* the ability to become financially independent, and *4)* the ability to independently form one's own beliefs and values. Very few participants believed that they had achieved these goals.

Data from the 2010 U.S. Census offer some supporting evidence regarding achievement of these important milestones. For example, more emerging adults are living with their parents than in the past (59% of males and 50% of females), with less than 5% living completely independently of their parents. In addition, the age of first marriage is getting older (from 22.5 years for men and 20.6 for women in 1970 to 28.4 for men and 26.5 for women in 2010). Given that today's youth do not assume more traditionally adult roles until their mid-to-late 20s, the assumption that individuals in this age-group are independent appears to be false. Therefore, it is a daunting challenge for pediatric clinics to successfully transfer the medical care of the emerging adult to adult providers. The adult medical system differs in its organization and integration of care from pediatric systems and all of this is occurring during the vulnerable stage of emerging adulthood. Not surprisingly, many young people hesitate to leave the familiarity, comfort, and security they have with their pediatric providers, especially during this critical phase of life. Similarly, it is not surprising that many pediatric providers worry about sending their patients into a different system of care that is less family-centered, and where multidisciplinary teams are less common.

Emerging adults with type 1 diabetes face a variety of challenges above and beyond the demands of the daily diabetes regimen. They are more independent of parental supervision and rules, but they must take on more responsibilities for self-care. They are learning how to find and keep a place to live, pay bills, balance their bank account records, manage credit, begin and keep a relationship that might be "forever," and pursue educational or career paths. All of these new tasks and goals are often negotiated at a time when emerging adults have less structure in their daily routine and less parental supervision and monitoring. For many emerging adults, these competing educational, economic, and social priorities detract from a focused commitment to the daily demands of diabetes care. Thus, programs focused on facilitating transition from pediatric to adult care have to provide developmentally appropriate health care in a coordinated, seamless manner across centers in partnerships with patients. The success of any transition program rests on both the pediatric and adult medical team's commitment to understanding emerging adults within this developmental context.

Transition Statistics and Outcomes

To meet such developmentally focused goals, medical teams must be able to distinguish between transition and transfer of care. Transition is not a one-time event. Instead, transition is a process that involves developing the skills necessary to be ready for adult life. In order for this process to be successful, transition planning must begin long before the actual transfer of care to an adult provider occurs. However, research demonstrates that programs transitioning adolescents and emerging adults with chronic illnesses to adult systems of care are poor or nonexistent, and patients are not well equipped to receive care in adult health care systems (Kipps 2002, Busse 2007, Gerstl 2008, Sparud-Lundin 2008, Helgeson 2009, Nakhla 2009, Petitti 2009). The National Survey of Children with Special Health Care Needs found that 60% of youth did not receive the services necessary to successfully transition from pediatric to adult care facilities.

It seems obvious that the health and well-being of teens and emerging adults with type 1 diabetes hinges on uninterrupted access to care, but data tell us reaching this goal is an uphill battle. First, there is a marked decline in clinic attendance around the time of transition: from 3.6 to 2.7 visits per year (Sparud-Lundin 2008). Second, among emerging adults with diabetes, 34% report a gap of greater than 6 months in establishing adult care (Garvey 2012) and approximately half of all adolescents and young adults with diabetes switch their adult care providers at least once after they leave their pediatric provider, resulting in delayed or missed medical care (Neu 2010).

Unfortunately, approximately 65% of youth with diabetes report at least one adverse medical outcome as a result of difficulties accessing medical care during the time of transition. Ironically, emerging adults seem to lose the care and support of a familiar medical system just when they most need that support. Gaps in care clearly result in poor metabolic control (Bryden 2001, Wills 2003), and this phenomenon is not unique to individuals living in the U.S. Worsening metabolic control has also been noted in longitudinal observational studies during the period of transitioning to adult care among youth living in a variety of countries (Sparud-Lundin 2008, Petitti 2009).

In addition to concerns about gaps in care as a result of difficulties accessing providers who work well with young people with type 1 diabetes, the period of transition from pediatric to adult care is also associated with an increase in short-term complications. For example, in a longitudinal study of more than 1,500 youth during the transition period, hospitalization rates increased from 7.6 to 9.5 per 100 patient years (Nakhla 2009). Long-term complications are first detected during this time of transition as well (Bryden 2001, Wills 2003). For example, one large study saw the prevalence of background retinopathy increase from 5% at 18 years of age to 29% at 24 years of age (Sparud-Lundin 2008), and another study reported that between 13% and 28% of emerging adults have nephropathy (Wills 2003). Above and beyond the increased risk for poor outcomes among emerging adults, research suggests that youth who are also ethnic minorities are at the greatest risk for poor health outcomes (Callahan 2001, Callahan 2010). This result is likely due to contextual variables from the environment, such as lower socioeconomic status, differences in health perceptions, and poorer access to health care. The collection of barriers to successful transition and optimal diabetes care characterizes these high-risk youth.

The need to address the worsening health outcomes among chronically ill youth has received some recognition among stakeholders and has led to the development of some disease-specific transition programming. Most of the literature on transition from pediatric to adult care is focused on the need for policy development, or on the need for physician training in the area of transitioning care (Callahan 2001, LoCasale-Crouch 2005). Studies evaluating illness-specific programs typically used retrospective research designs, focusing on issues such as patient satisfaction with the transfer process, patient recommendations about program changes that could improve the transfer process, or discomfort among adult care physicians in meeting the needs of youth with complex pediatric conditions. From the patient perspective, pediatric programs do not prepare them well for transition. Less than half of emerging adults report that their pediatric providers offered recommendations for adult providers (Garvey 2012), and less than 15% report that they participated in a transition-specific visit with their pediatric provider before leaving the pediatric practice (Garvey 2012).

Only two research teams have completed prospective evaluations of transition programs for youth with type 1 diabetes. The Maestro Project in Canada provided a project coordinator or *patient navigator* who maintained telephone and e-mail contact with emerging adults to provide support, identify barriers to accessing the adult diabetes system, and facilitate communication among patients and providers as well as community resources. The program also sponsored a casual evening drop-in group every 4–6 weeks and occasional educational events. Results show a decline in no-show rates from 25% to 35% down to 11%. Similarly, Holmes-Walker (2007) in Australia created a transition coordinator position to work with their emerging adult population. They developed a young adult diabetes clinic in the adult hospital, located adjacent to the pediatric hospital. Their coordinator offered appointment reminders and appointment rebooking for their emerging adults. The program also offered after-hours support for sick days. Findings suggest that A1C levels improved if at least two clinic appointments were attended in the first year. They also found a decrease in DKA admissions among program participants. Both of these studies suggest that emerging adults respond well to having an easily reachable point person who can help them navigate the adult system.

Given the high risk that chronically ill youth face during the vulnerable time of transitioning from pediatric to adult care, surprisingly little evidence-based research exists to guide the development of empirically based interventions aimed at improving transition services, access to care, and health outcomes. There is a great need for empirical evidence describing factors that facilitate or inhibit successful transitions. However, the current transitions literature can still guide health care professionals in creating a developmentally appropriate road map for facilitating a successful transfer of care from a pediatric to an adult provider for patients with diabetes. The consensus report published by the American Academy of Pediatrics, the American Academy of Family Physicians, and the American College of Physicians in 2011 offers a practice-based guide for implementing transition services for youth with chronic illness.

The Four-Step Process

According to the consensus report mentioned above, transition planning should be completed via a four-step process and should begin early, to allow time for the patient to develop and build the necessary skills for a successful transition process. In the first step, initiated when the patient is between the ages of 11 and 12 years, the health care provider should sit down with the patient and family members to review the program's formal transition policy. This written policy should include the following information:

1. The expected age of patient transfer to adult care (some programs expect individuals to transfer during high school, some at the end of high school, some at the end of the college).
2. The patient's responsibilities for preparing for transition.
3. Parental responsibilities for preparing for transition.
4. The medical team's responsibilities for preparing for transition.

The goal of this first step is to raise a family's awareness of future goals and get everyone thinking about life after high school. This first step in the transition process coincides with the time when many pediatricians begin to spend a few minutes alone with their patients, giving these patients the experience of talking directly with their provider, and helping them begin to develop the communication, advocacy, and self-care skills necessary for a successful transfer of care in the future. This brief patient-only time also begins preparing parents for eventually trusting that their children have the skills necessary to manage their own health care (American Academy of Pediatrics 2008).

In the second step of the transition process, the medical team and the family should jointly develop a formalized and individualized transition plan. This step should occur when the patient is around 14 years of age, which is also the start of high school. This formalized plan should acknowledge the patient's current abilities and responsibilities as well as the family members' abilities and responsibilities. Often, the formalized plan is based on an assessment of the adolescent's skills, abilities, and responsibilities via a checklist. Once the medical team and family agree on where the teenager's skills are, goals for achieving increased skills, abilities, and independent responsibilities should be discussed and mutually agreed upon.

Our clinical experience suggests that facilitating transition involves more than assessing specific skill sets. Developing a sense of comfort in talking openly with health care providers about personal and intimate issues is a vital skill for successful adult care. We encourage providers to use this time to engage in open discussions with their teenage patients about their sexual activity, condom use and other safe sex practices, and the need for preconception counseling. Discussions about the impact of alcohol on blood glucose levels and ways to drink safely are also important to have during the high school years. Similarly, issues related to driving safely should be brought up during these private conversations.

In the third step of the transition process, the medical team, the adolescent, and family members should review the transition plan annually, assess the goals that have been achieved since the last visit, and assess and problem solve around barriers to achieving the remaining goals. This third step occurs between the ages of 15 and 17 years. We encourage clinicians to make sure that the parents review their child's insurance coverage during this time. Some changes in access to insurance occur between the ages of 18 and 21 years, while others do not change until 26 years of age, and families need to understand these changes before they occur. There are a number of already-published checklists to guide goal achievement (see Figures 10.1 and 10.2).

Finally, in the fourth step of the transition process, which occurs between the ages of 18 and 21 years, the patient would either transfer to an adult provider or the pediatric team would implement an adult model of care while working with the patient. One of the goals for this phase is the development of a portable medical summary. Ideally, this summary would be created jointly

FIGURE 10.1. USEFUL WEBSITES FOR MANAGING THE TRANSITION PROCESS

- http://www.gottransition.org
- http://illinoisaap.org/projects/medical-home/transition/resources-for-physicians
- http://www.dragonflyheartcamp.org/retreat%20facts/assets/transitionreadinessquestionaire.pdf
- https://www.luriechildrens.org/en-us/care-services/specialties-services/transitioning-to-adult-care/planning/Pages/community_resources.aspx
- http://www.jaxHATS.ufl.edu/docs
- http://www.sickkids.ca/good2go
- http://www.diabetes.org/assets/pdfs/schools/going-to-college-with-diabetes.pdf (a self-advocacy guide offered by the American Diabetes Association)
- CollegeDiabetesNetwork.org (a website offering peer support, information, and resources to youth attending college)

by the patient and the provider. During this time a list of possible adult care providers would be given to the patient, who would schedule initial visits with at least one adult provider.

FIGURE 10.2. DIABETES SKILLS CHECKLIST

		Someone else always does this for me	I do not do this by myself often, but I am starting to try	I sometimes do this by myself, and sometimes some-one else does it for me	I usually do this by myself, but sometimes someone else helps me	I always do this by myself
INSULIN						
1	I take my insulin without anyone reminding me					
2	I know when the insulin(s) I'm taking peak in my body					
3	I know how long the insulin(s) I'm taking last in my body					
4	I adjust my insulin dose based on my blood sugar readings					
5	I adjust my insulin based on carbohydrate counting					
6	I adjust my insulin based on how much I exercise					
BLOOD SUGARS						
1	I check my blood sugars without being reminded to					
2	I use my blood sugar numbers to identify patterns					
3	I use my blood sugar numbers to determine my dose of insulin					
4	I use my blood sugar numbers to determine if it is safe to drive					
5	I use my blood sugar numbers to decide if I have successfully treated a low					

		Someone else always does this for me	I do not do this by myself often, but I am starting to try	I sometimes do this by myself, and sometimes someone else does it for me	I usually do this by myself, but sometimes someone else helps me	I always do this by myself
HYPOGLYCEMIA						
1	I keep supplies for treating lows with me at all times					
CARBOHYDRATES/FOODS						
1	I can accurately count carbohydrates in my foods					
2	I can accurately judge portion sizes					
3	I can read food labels					
4	I know how many carbohydrates are in my beverages					
EXERCISE						
1	I check blood sugars before I begin to exercise					
2	I keep supplies for treating lows with me when I exercise					
3	I check blood sugars two hours after exercise					
ACTION PLANS						
1	I know how to fill my prescriptions (insulin, syringes, pump supplies, strips)					
2	I know what my insurance coverage is for my prescriptions					
3	I pay for my prescriptions					
4	I order my supplies before I run out					
5	I know how to make an appointment with members of my diabetes team					
6	I know how to contact members of my diabetes team if I have questions or want to talk with them					
7	I am comfortable talking with my diabetes team about my own care					
8	I know how to handle sick days					

Case Example

Marissa is a 17-year-old junior in high school who has lived with type 1 diabetes since she was 9 years old. Her pediatric diabetes team shared their transition policy with her and her parents when she was 12 years old. They discussed the goal of helping her develop the skills needed to leave home and go away to college, and they talked about having 6 full years to build those skills. Twice each year, Marissa and her parents reviewed her self-care skills with the members of her diabetes team, who developed plans for her to slowly increase her confidence in what she could do, while still maintaining the support of her parents. Initially, Marissa was hesitant to take on some of these skills, but she felt relieved to know that nothing needed to be changed quickly. There were times when she felt very overwhelmed (applying for a competitive high school; trying out for the sophomore debate team; breaking up with her first boyfriend) and asked her parents to take over her diabetes care. After a while, Marissa felt she was ready to take back the responsibility for her own care. After that, to help decrease her sense of being overwhelmed, Marissa and her parents downloaded her blood glucose and her pump information each Sunday evening and looked for patterns so that they could problem solve together.

As Marissa got older, her understanding of "insulin on board," her ability to make decisions regarding her insulin-to-carbohydrate ratios, and her basal rates all improved. She now monitors her own supplies and calls her pharmacy to renew prescriptions before they run out. She called her team's hotline number when her pump failed last month, and she also calls them to guide her when she's had strep. Her diabetes team members continue to see their patients through the college years, so Marissa feels good about maintaining a close relationship with them while she negotiates life in a dorm. Her parents have promised her that they will not move into the dorm with her.

11
Advocacy

Wouldn't it be amazing if all of your adolescent patients became advocates in the area of diabetes? Can you imagine each of your patients choosing diabetes as a personal mission? Well, it is possible. It is an achievable goal.

Adolescents work for causes that are important to them (getting a driver's license, or getting their curfew bumped up to midnight, or getting the newest video game, or getting accepted to the college of their choice). The question is whether or not you can help your patients choose diabetes as an important cause. Your patients may choose to be their own advocates—they may wish to learn how to tell you what they need, and what aspects of diabetes are difficult and annoying for them. They may wish to learn how to communicate more effectively with their parents about diabetes-specific issues. They may wish to become more comfortable talking with their friends or romantic partners about diabetes.

In addition, you may find that some of your patients are interested in working to advocate for the broader community of people with diabetes. Perhaps your patients want to work on fund-raising, on finding a cure, on improving access to health care services, on improving access to technology and devices for those who struggle with insurance coverage, or on protecting the rights of people with diabetes. Any advocacy mission, no matter what it may be, teaches our patients important life lessons.

Learning the skills necessary for getting what they want and what they need is an important developmental goal for adolescents. Some adolescents seem particularly skilled at getting what they want (designer clothes, the newest footwear, concert tickets), others less so. Helping your patients develop advocacy skills around diabetes issues provides them with real-world experience that they can use in a variety of areas of their life both now and in the future. As a member of a diabetes team, one of your core duties is to teach, and what greater reward can there be than seeing your patients become teachers as well? Helping your adolescent patients advocate for their own needs with their diabetes team, their parents, and their peers—or advocate for the larger diabetes community—not only meets your mission as a teacher, but also serves as a terrific advocacy goal for yourself.

Helping Teenagers Advocate for Their Own Diabetes Needs

With their health care team (that's you!). Talk directly to your adolescent patients, and let them know that you are interested in hearing their thoughts, ideas, and questions. This promotes an environment of open communication, which is critical for being an advocate. Let them know that you do not have all the answers, and acknowledge that diabetes is an incredibly frustrating disease. Acknowledge that what they do each day does not always show up in the numbers they see on their blood glucose meter. Acknowledge that puberty can cause wacky blood glucose numbers—as can growing, stress, and things we do not know how to measure yet. If you do not have diabetes yourself, let them know you recognize that as much as you might try, you will never really know what it is like to live with diabetes.

Let them know that you see them as the experts on their own diabetes— what works for them and what does not work for them. Acknowledge that whatever they think or feel about diabetes is right—because it's *their* diabetes. Let them know that you want to partner with them in their journey through diabetes. Let them know that you can be a member of their team only if they are open and honest with you. Invite them to let you know when they think you are not understanding them, or when they feel you are judging them. Invite them to let you know when they have questions that they may find embarrassing or awkward.

One easy way to teach your patients to become advocates for th
is to ask them, each and every time you see them, what questions they want
answered during this visit, or what frustrations they'd like to overcome during
this visit. At each visit, help your patients set small, achievable, concrete, and
specific goals that are important to them. Each of the recommendations we
have listed above will help teach your patients how to advocate for their own
health care needs, both with you and with other providers they will meet along
the way.

With their parents. One of the key developmental tasks of adolescence
is separating from parents and becoming an individual able to independently
form opinions, ideas, and goals (Arnett 2010). Adolescents are interested in
becoming more independent from their parents, and independence in diabetes care is part of that. However, adherence to the diabetes regimen declines
as parental supervision declines (DiMatteo 2002, Busse 2007, Helgeson 2009,
Petitti 2009). Once adherence declines, parent-adolescent conflict increases.
Most teenagers perceive this conflict as caused by parent intrusiveness, parent
nagging, or parent disrespect. Only rarely do teenagers see parent nagging as
an expression of worry, concern, and love. However, you—the health care provider—can help your adolescent patients hear their parents' nagging as expres-
sions of worry and concern, and you can also teach your adolescent patients
how to advocate for themselves without increasing family conflict.

Why is it important to teach your patients these skills? Because the data on
family conflict during adolescence are clear, consistent, and compelling: ado-
lescent-parent conflict is associated with worse adherence (Anderson 2002,
Weibe 2005, Ellis 2008b, Helgeson 2009, Weissberg-Benchell 2009, Wysocki
2009, Ingerski 2010, Hilliard 2011), worse metabolic control (Anderson 2002,
Weibe 2005, Hood 2007, Ellis 2008b, Helgeson 2009, Weissberg-Benchell
2009, Williams 2009, Wysocki 2009, Ingerski 2010, Hilliard 2011), worse
quality of life (Weissberg-Benchel 2009, Wysocki 2009), and increased depressive symptoms (Williams 2009, Wysocki 2009). OK, so you now have research
data to confirm what you already know clinically: parent-adolescent conflict is
not good for either diabetes or psychosocial outcomes. So how do you teach
your patients ways to advocate for themselves while also reducing conflict?

Sometimes, the conflict is really only about figuring out who is responsible
for what aspects of the diabetes regimen. So it may be helpful to ask these

questions of the parent and the adolescent while they are both in the room together:

Who is responsible for insulin administration in the morning? Afternoon? Evening? Snacking?

Who is responsible for pattern management decisions?

Who is in charge of ordering meter supplies?

Who takes care of pump site changes or making sure injection sites are rotated?

Who is supposed to tell teachers/coaches/other adults about diabetes?

Sometimes this conversation reveals that no one is responsible; assumptions about responsibility were made that led to misunderstanding and conflict. Helping families talk openly about and negotiate expectations and responsibilities teaches your patients how to advocate for themselves with their parents and also reduces parent-child conflict.

Sometimes the source of conflict is a result of what Anderson and Coyne termed *miscarried helping*. Miscarried helping was discussed in the chapter on parent-teen relationships; as a reminder, it occurs when parents are worried or concerned about their adolescent's choices and behaviors around diabetes care. They express that concern in a manner that is perceived as anything but supportive or concerned. In fact, the adolescent only hears nagging ("Why are your blood glucose levels so high? What did you eat?" or "You forgot to bolus again, didn't you?" or "Do you want to go blind by the time you're 30?" or "Did you check your blood glucose? Are you sure you checked your blood glucose? I don't see your numbers!").

These blaming comments are also seen by the adolescents as accusations by their parents that they are irresponsible and incompetent. Once the adolescent feels blamed, accused, and untrustworthy, their desire to collaborate with their parents around diabetes concerns is severely and negatively impacted. Once teenagers expect such parental reactions, they are not very likely to reach out to their parents to help them problem solve around bolusing for a Frappuccino™ or a Slurpee®. They are not very likely to talk openly and honestly with their parents about the days when their numbers are running high no matter what they do to correct them. After a while, the communication between parent and teenager becomes less frequent and everyone becomes increasingly angry and frustrated with each other. This leads to parents feeling even more worried and concerned about their child's health and safety, and the vicious cycle of miscarried helping continues. It is important to recognize that miscarried helping can happen to anyone, and is not a sign of psychopathology. It happens because people love and care about each other and want their loved ones to be safe and healthy.

If you suspect that miscarried helping is the source of family conflict for any of your patients, there is actually a fairly straightforward way to teach these patients how to advocate for themselves with their parents and decrease conflict at the same time. This strategy can be used during any clinic visit and should not take more than about 10 minutes. When you have the adolescent and the parent in the room together, turn to the teenager and ask: "Can you guess how many hours a day your parents nag you about diabetes things?" Most teenagers will guess a minimum of 8 hours in a day. Sometimes they may even say 14 or more hours, implying that their parents go to school with them or sleep in their bedroom. It is important to accept any amount of time, as this is about understanding adolescent perception, not uncovering facts.

Once you get an answer, ask: "How many minutes a day do you need to do all of your diabetes care (like checking blood glucose, taking insulin, counting carbs, changing infusion sets)?" Please notice that we asked about HOURS of nagging and MINUTES of diabetes regimen tasks. Next, juxtapose the hours with the minutes by saying something like: "Twenty minutes of diabetes tasks and 8 hours of nagging. That's not such a good deal. It must seem like your parents wake up and think, 'What can we do to annoy our son today? Oh, let's nag him about diabetes.' But I'll bet that doesn't actually happen." Your patient will very likely tell you that he or she knows for a fact that his or her parents spend their time plotting and planning various ways of annoying him or her. You may wish to respond by saying something like: "I know that most parents nag by accident. They mean to say, 'We're worried about you. We want you to be safe.' They're not sure you're doing what is needed to stay healthy." Then turn to the parents and ask them: "Do you enjoy nagging? Is it fun?" Most parents will clearly state that they can't stand it.

The next step in this intervention strategy is to point out that the two sides are not communicating effectively. You might choose to do that by saying something like: "Natalie hears nagging, but you're trying to tell her you're worried for her safety and health. I'd like to ask all of you for permission to try an experiment that may help the nagging go away AND keep Natalie safe."

Then ask the family to try this experiment for only 2 weeks. (Two weeks is a reasonable time frame that will minimize frustration if the experiment does not go well initially.) Let the family know that this experiment can only take place when the adolescent and parent are in the same place. It can't work when the teen is at school or a friend's home.

Next, look directly at the teenager and say something like: "Natalie, when it's time to check your blood glucose, take insulin, change an infusion set, count carbs, correct lows, or do other diabetes-related tasks, and your parents are around, you must do these tasks in front of them. As long as these tasks are done in front of them, no matter what happens, your parents can't say a word about diabetes—no questions, no comments, nothing." Then turn to face the parents and say something like: "Natalie is sacrificing her privacy in order to help you feel more comfortable that she's doing things safely. So, you won't need to nag her, since you'll see she's done what's necessary." Finally, turn to the adolescent and say something like: "Natalie, this means you'll save 8 hours of nagging, but lose about 20 minutes of privacy. It's 8 hours versus 20 minutes."

Typically, adolescents are convinced that their parents will not be able to keep their word. Let your patient know it's good to be skeptical. Also remind your patient that since it's an experiment, you don't know whether this plan will work or not. If possible, schedule a clinic follow-up visit or a phone call to review the family's progress in 2 weeks' time. Our experience is that this strategy is remarkably successful.

With their friends. Adolescents spend more time with their friends than they do with their parents. Therefore, helping them learn how to advocate for themselves while they're with their friends is an important goal. Friends can offer a significant amount of emotional support and facilitate an adolescent's ability to cope with diabetes (Bearman 2002, Wysocki 2006). In fact, teens who perceived empathy and support from their friends showed better adherence and greater emotional well-being (Malik 2012). In addition, teens report that having friends remind them to engage in self-care tasks is helpful (Lehmkuhl 2009). Talking with your patients about their friendships and how they talk with their friends about diabetes is an important topic of conversation and will help your adolescent patients learn to become effective advocates for themselves.

One way to help your patients is to ask them whom they have told about their diabetes. If they have pretty much kept their diabetes to themselves, then this is an area that will require ongoing conversation. Teens who are secretive about their diabetes tend to engage in less self-care and have worse metabolic control. They are also more overwhelmed by their disease and less able to advocate for their needs.

If you have patients who are keeping their diabetes secret, then it is important to explore what their fears and concerns are. Are they afraid that they'll have to answer too many personal questions? Are they afraid that people will reject them or think they're contagious? Perhaps they just do not want to be different from their peers. It is important to discuss these worries and concerns and to address them directly. Typically, helping your patients come up with one or two answers to the most likely questions is helpful—so that they have answers at the ready. Work with your patients on developing concrete answers about diabetes, such as: "My body doesn't make insulin so I have to replace it with an injection (or through my pump)," or "I can eat anything as long as I count my carbohydrates and cover them with insulin." Or "Yup, I have type 1 diabetes, which can be annoying sometimes, but by taking care of it, I can do anything I want to do."

For those patients who are comfortable talking about diabetes with their friends, it may be helpful to ask those patients what aspects of diabetes their friends currently support and what ways their friends can be even more supportive. For example, some teens find that having their friends text them during lunch with a reminder to bolus is helpful. Some find that teaching carb counting to a close friend is helpful. Some find that the most important skill a friend can have is the ability to recognize and treat lows (especially when alcohol is involved).

Finally, although it may be an uncomfortable topic to discuss, our teenagers are thinking about romantic relationships all the time. Ask your patients about how and when they talk about their diabetes with a girlfriend or boyfriend. They may have questions about technology and sex (e.g., "How long can I disconnect from the pump when I'm having sex?" or "How do I explain that my CGM will not pop off during sex?"). Inviting your teen patients to talk with you about these questions is an important step in teaching them how to advocate for themselves when they are faced with romantic-partner issues. Of course, it is also vital to talk with your female patients about preconception counseling (Charron-Prochownik 2008, Fischl 2010) to help them advocate for their own reproductive health. This was covered in more detail in the chapter on high-risk behaviors.

Helping Teenagers Advocate for the Larger Diabetes Community

Adolescents are very often willing to work hard for a cause that is important to them. Working for the greater good gives them an appreciation for what they already have, allows them to see that there is more to the world than just their own circle of family and friends, and provides a means for connecting with the world. Teens who volunteer learn a sense of commitment to their society. They learn vital leadership skills such as communication, teamwork, negotiating, and organization. Volunteering also offers them a sense of ownership and pride in the work that they do and the effort they put forth. You can help your adolescent patients become advocates in the world of diabetes by letting them know about the many volunteer opportunities available.

Advocacy through the American Diabetes Association (www.diabetes.org/advocate)

The Association offers advocacy experiences in the areas of school safety, insurance coverage, research toward a cure, legal support around discrimination issues, and public accommodations (e.g., being able to take diabetes supplies into theaters and stadiums and through airport security). Teenagers can apply to become the Association's National Youth Advocate. The advocate spends one year spreading awareness and advocating for people with diabetes through public speaking. The advocate testifies before the U.S. Congress to promote the Association's legislative priorities. The selected teen attends diabetes conferences and diabetes camps, and works to motivate others to make a difference in the lives of those with diabetes.

Teens have probably experienced frustrating situations at school involving diabetes care. The Association's Safe at Schools campaign is focused on ensuring that students with diabetes are medically safe and have access to the same educational opportunities as their peers. So far, laws have been passed in 17 states. Your patients may be able to work with their local chapter of the Association and their state legislators to help get the legislation passed in all 50 states.

The Association's antidiscrimination work may also be of interest to your adolescent patients. Since discrimination typically stems from ignorance, helping your patients learn the skills necessary to teach others about diabetes will reduce ignorance and thereby, hopefully, reduce discrimination. In fact, the American Diabetes Association's philosophy on addressing discrimination is to first Educate, then Negotiate, then Litigate, and finally Legislate.

The Association also offers a website just for youth with diabetes, Planet D (http://www.diabetes.org/living-with-diabetes/parents-and-kids/planet-d).

Advocacy through the JDRF
(www.jdrf.org)

The JDRF offers advocacy experiences aimed at curing, treating, and preventing type 1 diabetes. Teenagers can get involved in supporting the JDRF's advocacy work with Congress to maintain funding for the two parts of the Special Diabetes Program: one part advances type 1 diabetes research at the National Institutes of Health (NIH), and the other funds treatment, education, and prevention programs for American Indian and Alaska Native populations, who are disproportionately affected by type 2 diabetes.

The JDRF also focuses on the artificial pancreas, which combines a continuous glucose monitor and insulin pump with sophisticated computer software to provide just the right amount of insulin at just the right time. The organization also advocates for stem cell research, health care reform, and diabetes management in schools. Finally, teenagers can get involved in JDRF's biannual Children's Congress, which brings teens and their families to Washington, DC, to meet with their members of Congress and congressional staff. Finally, JDRF has great resources just for teenagers at http://jdrf.org/life-with-t1d/teenagers.

Advocacy through social networking

Your teen patients use social media every single day. Why not encourage them to engage in advocacy via social media?

Children with Diabetes (*www.childrenwithdiabetes.com*). This website was started by Jeff Hitchcock after his young daughter was diagnosed with type 1 diabetes. It is one of the most popular websites for families, children, teenagers, and adults dealing with diabetes. In addition to providing online information and offering communication forums, Children with Diabetes promotes the "Quilt for Life" diabetes awareness project, and hosts Friends for Life conferences to provide education and support for youth with diabetes and their families.

Type 1 Nation (*www.typeonenation.org*). This social networking site was created for and by people with type 1 diabetes and their loved ones. It was launched by JDRF on World Diabetes Day, November 14, 2008. Type 1 Nation is open to anyone over the age of 13 years.

dLife (*www.dLife.com*). This website's goal is to promote education and motivation for people with diabetes, particularly children with diabetes, in order to empower them to take control and live a long, healthy life. The dLife Foundation supports individuals who need diabetes supplies, education, and motivational programs, through organizations, foundations, and camps.

Close Concerns (*www.closeconcerns.com*). This website offers an online newsletter (diaTribe; www.diaTribe.us) that reports on new research and products for people with diabetes. It offers information and insights from others with diabetes as well as opinions about what is available to the diabetes community.

Diabetes Hands Foundation (*www.diabeteshandsfoundation.org*). This online foundation provides a place for people with diabetes and their loved ones to connect and have an open dialogue about their experiences with this chronic condition. Diabetes Hands Foundation seeks to understand, connect, and energize the millions of people living with this condition. The foundation sponsors two online communities: TuDiabetes (www.tudiabetes.org) for English-speaking individuals and EsTuDiabetes (www.Estudiabetes.org) for Spanish-speaking individuals. Both communities offer a culturally sensitive experience to their members, helping them connect with others they can relate to.

Six Until Me (*www.sixuntilme.com*). This blog is written by Kerri Sparling, who believes strongly in the power of sharing diabetes stories with others. She helps people with diabetes feel that they are not alone with this disease. She does so with honesty and humor.

Scottsdiabetes (*www.scottsdiabetes.com*). This blog is written by Scott Johnson. He and Kerri Sparling were among the first bloggers on living with diabetes. In the years since Scott and Kerri began blogging, the diabetes online community has become ever larger. Scott feels strongly that the support and encouragement he finds from the online community plays a crucial role in his well-being. Scott may not be giving himself enough credit for all he does to help others who read his blog.

Diabetes Mine (*www.diabetesmine.com*). This blog site was created by and for patients as a "diabetes newspaper with a personal twist." The site provides news, research updates, and product reviews, and encourages guest posts.

Bibliography

American Academy of Pediatrics: *Bright Futures: Guidelines for Health Supervision of Infants, Children and Adolescents.* 3rd ed. Hagen J, Shaw J, Duncan P (Eds). Elk Grove, IL, American Academy of Pediatrics, 2008

American Academy of Pediatrics, American Academy of Family Physicians, American College of Physicians: Consensus statement: supporting the health care transition from adolescence to adulthood in the medical home. *Pediatrics* 128:182–200, 2011

American Diabetes Association: Standards of medical care in diabetes—2009. *Diabetes Care* 32 (Suppl. 1):S13–S61, 2009

Anderson BJ: Family conflict and diabetes management in youth: clinical lessons from child development and diabetes research. *Diabetes Spectrum* 17:22–26, 2004

Anderson BJ, Vangsness L, Connell A, Butler D, Goebel-Fabbri A, Laffel L: Family conflict, adherence, and glycaemic control in youth with short duration type 1 diabetes. *Diabet Med* 19:635–642, 2002

Anderson BJ, Rubin RR: *Practical Psychology for Diabetes Clinicians: How to Deal with the Key Behavioral Issues Faced by Patients and Health Care Teams.* Alexandria, VA, American Diabetes Association, 1996

Anderson BJ, Coyne JC: "Miscarried helping" in the families of children and adolescents with chronic diseases. In *Advances in Child Health Psychology,* Johnson JH, Johnson SB, Eds. Gainesville, FL, University of Florida Press, 1991, p. 167–177

Arnett JJ: *Adolescence and Emerging Adulthood: A Cultural Approach.* 4th ed. Boston, MA, Prentice-Hall, 2010

Arnett JJ: *Emerging Adulthood: The Winding Road from the Late Teens through the Twenties.* New York, Oxford University Press, 2004

Arnett JJ: Emerging adulthood. A theory of development from the late teens through the twenties. *Am Psychol* 55:469–480, 2000

Arnett, JJ: Adolescent storm and stress, reconsidered. *Am Psychol* 54:317–325, 1999

Ashton M: The dangers of warnings. *Drug and Alcohol Findings* 1:22–24, 1999

Baldassano R, Ferry G, Griffiths A, Mack D, Markowitz J, Winter H: Transition of the patient with inflammatory bowel disease from pediatric to adult care: recommendations of the North American Society for Pediatric Gastroenterology, Hepatology and Nutrition. *J Pediatr Gastroenterol Nutr* 34:245–248, 2002

Bearman KJ, LaGreca A: Assessing friend support of adolescents' diabetes care: the diabetes social support questionnaire—friends version. *J Pediatr Psychol* 27:417–428, 2002

Bell L, Sawyer S: Transition of care to adult services for pediatric solid-organ transplant recipients. *Pediatr Clin North Am* 57:593–610, 2010

Bell L, Bartosh S, Davis C, Dobbels F, Al-Uzri A, Lotstein D, Reiss J: Adolescent transition to adult care in solid organ transplantation: a consensus conference report. *Am J Transplant* 8:2230–2242, 2008

Bronfrenbrenner U: *The Ecology of Human Development: Experiments by Nature and Design.* Cambridge, MA, Harvard University Press, 1979

Bryden KS, Peveler RC, Stein A, Neil A, Mayou RA, Dunger DB: Clinical and psychological course of diabetes from adolescence to young adulthood. *Diabetes Care* 24:1536–1540, 2001

Busse F, Hiermann P, Galler A, Stumvoll M, Wiessner T, Kiess W, Kapellen T: Evaluation of patients' opinion and glycemic control after transfer of young adults with type 1 diabetes from a pediatric diabetes clinic to adult care. *Horm Res* 67:132–138, 2007

Callahan ST, Cooper WO: Changes in ambulatory health care use during the transition to young adulthood. *J Adolesc Health* 46:407–413, 2010

Callahan S, Winitzer R, Keenan P: Transition from pediatric to adult-oriented health care: a challenge for patients with chronic disease. *Curr Opin Pediatr* 13:310–316, 2001

Centers for Disease Control and Prevention: Youth risk behavior surveillance—United States—2009. *Morbidity and Mortality Weekly Report Surveillance Summary.* 59(ss-5), 2010

Charron-Prochownik D, Ferons-Hannan M, Sereika S, Becker D: Randomized efficacy trial of early preconception counseling for diabetic teens (READY-girls). *Diabetes Care* 31:1327–1330, 2008

Colton PA, Olmsted MP, Daneman D, Rydall AC, Rodin GM: Natural history and predictors of disturbed eating behaviour in girls with type 1 diabetes. *Diabet Med* 24:424–429, 2007

Corathers S, Kichler J, Jones NH, Houchen A, Jolly M, Morwessel N, Crawford P, Dolan L, Hood KK: Improving depression screening for adolescents with type 1 diabetes. *Pediatrics* 2013 October 14 [Epub ahead of print]

Cox DJ, Kovatchev BP, Anderson SM, Clarke WL, Gonder-Frederick L: Type 1 diabetic drivers with and without a history of recurrent hypoglycemia-related driving mishaps: physiological and performance differences during euglycemia and the induction of hypoglycemia. *Diabetes Care* 33:2430–2435, 2010

Cox DJ, Ford D, Gonder-Frederick L, Clarke W, Mazze R, Weinger K, Ritterbrand L: Driving mishaps among individuals with type 1 diabetes: a prospective study. *Diabetes Care* 32:2177–2180, 2009

Cox DJ, Penberthy JK, Zrebiec J, et al.: Diabetes and driving mishaps: frequency and correlations from a multinational survey. *Diabetes Care* 26:2329–2334, 2003

Cox DJ, Gonder-Frederick L, Kovatchev BP, Julian DM, Clarke WL: Progressive hypoglycemia's impact on driving simulation performance: occurrence, awareness and correction. *Diabetes Care* 23:163–170, 2000

DiMatteo M, Giordani P, Lepper H, Croghan T: Patient adherence and medical treatment outcomes: a meta-analysis. *Medical Care* 40:794–811, 2002

Ellis D, Naar-King S, Templin T, Frey M, Cunningham P, Sheidow A, Idalski A: Multisystemic therapy for adolescents with poorly controlled type 1 diabetes: reduced diabetic ketoacidosis admissions and related costs over 24 months. *Diabetes Care* 31:1746–1747, 2008a

Ellis D, Templin T, Podolski C, Frey M, Naar-King S, Moltz K: The parent monitoring of diabetes care scale: development, reliability and validity of a scale to evaluate parental supervision of adolescent illness management. *J Adolesc Health* 42:146–152, 2008b

Feltbower RG, Bodansky HJ, Patterson CC, Parslow RC, Stephenson CR, Reynolds C, McKinney PA: Acute complications and drug misuse are important causes of death for children and young adults with type 1 diabetes: results from the Yorkshire register of diabetes in children and young adults. *Diabetes Care* 31:922–926, 2008

Fischl AF, Herman WH, Sereika SM, Hannan M, Becker D, Mansfield MJ, Freytag LL, Milaszewski K, Botscheller AN, Charron-Prochownik D: Impact of a preconception counseling program for teens with type 1 diabetes (READY-Girls) on patient-provider interaction, resource utilization, and cost. *Diabetes Care* 33:701–705, 2010

Fishbein M, Hall-Jamieson K, Zimmer E, von Haeften I, Nabi R: Avoiding the boomerang: testing the relative effectiveness of antidrug public service announcements before a national campaign. *Am J Public Health* 92:238–245, 2002

Garvey KC, Wolpert HA, Rhodes ET, et al.: Health care transition in patients with type 1 diabetes: young adult experiences and relationship to glycemic control. *Diabetes Care* 35:1716–1722, 2012

Gerstl E, Rabl W, Rosenbauer J, Grobe H, Hofer S, Krause U, Holl R: Glycemic control as reflected by HbA1c in children, adolescents and young adults with type 1 diabetes mellitus: combined longitudinal analysis including 27,035 patients from 207 centers in Germany and Austria during the last decade. *Eur J Pediatr* 167:447–453, 2008

Goebel-Fabbri AE, Fikkan J, Franko DL, Pearson K, Anderson BJ, Weinger K: Insulin restriction and associated morbidity and mortality in women with type 1 diabetes mellitus. *Diabetes Care* 31:415–417, 2008

Griffin SJ, Kinmonth AL, Veitman MW, Gillard S, Grant J, Stewart M: Effect on health-related outcomes of interventions to alter the interactions between patients and practitioners: a systematic review of trials. *Ann Fam Med* 2:595–608, 2004

Haidt J: *The Happiness Hypothesis: Finding Modern Truth in Ancient Wisdom.* New York, Basic Books, 2006

Hall GS: *Adolescence: Its Psychology and Its Relation to Physiology, Anthropology, Sociology, Sex, Crime, Religion, and Education.* Vols. I and II. Englewood Cliffs, NJ, Prentice-Hall, 1904

Harris MA, Spiro K, Heywood M, Hatten A, Hoehn D, Wagner MA: Piloting intensive behavioral health for youth with T1DM: avoiding avoidable hospitalizations [Abstract]. *Diabetes* 73:827-P, 2013a

Harris MA, Spiro K, Heywood M, Wagner D, Hoehn D, Hatten A, Labby D: Novel interventions in children's health care (NICH): innovative treatment for youth with complex medical conditions. *Clin Pract Pediatr Psychol* 1:137–145, 2013b

Harris MA, Freeman KA, Duke DC, Hirschfield B, Boston B: Can you hear (and see) me now?: Skype-based intervention for teens with poorly controlled diabetes [Abstract]. *Diabetes* 72:345-OR, 2012a

Harris MA, Hood KK, Mulvaney SA: Pumpers, skypers, surfers, and texters: technology to improve the management of diabetes in teenagers. *Diabetes Obes Metab* 14:967–972, 2012b

Harris MA, Raymond JK, Duke DC: Optimizing transitional care for emerging adults with type 1 diabetes: what needs to be done and by whom? *Diabetes Management* 2:269–271, 2012c

Harris MA, Freeman KA, Duke DC: Transitioning from pediatric to adult health care: dropping off the face of the earth. *Am J Lifestyle Med* 5:85–91, 2011

Harris MA, Antal H, Oelbaum R, Buckloh LM, White NH, Wysocki T: Good intentions gone awry: assessing parental miscarried helping in diabetes. *Fam Syst Health* 26:393–403, 2008

Harris MA: Dogs, cats, and diabetes. *Diabetes Spectrum* 19:187–189, 2006

Harris MA, Mertlich D: Piloting home-based behavioral family systems therapy for adolescents with poorly controlled diabetes. *Child Health Care* 32:65–79, 2003

Harris MA, Mertlich D, Rothweiler J: Parenting the child with diabetes. *Diabetes Spectrum* 14:182–184, 2001

Health Resources and Service Administration, Maternal and Child Health Bureau: The National Survey of Children with Special Health Care Needs Chartbook 2005–2006. Rockville, MD, U.S. Department of Health and Human Services, Health Resources and Service Administration, Maternal and Child Health Bureau, 2008

Helgeson V, Siminerio L, Escobar O, Becker D: Predictors of glycemic control among adolescents with diabetes: a 4-year longitudinal study. *J Pediatr Psychol* 34:254–270, 2009

Hilliard ME, Monaghan M, Cogen FR, Streisand R: Parent stress and child behaviour among young children with type 1 diabetes. *Child Care Health Dev* 37:224–32, 2011

Holmes-Walker DJ, Llewellyn AC, Farrell K: A transition care programme which improves diabetes control and reduces hospital admission rates in young adults with type 1 diabetes aged 15-25 years. *Diabet Med* 24:764–769, 2007

Hood K, Butler D, Anderson B, Laffel L: Updated and revised Diabetes Family Conflict Scale. *Diabetes Care* 30:1764–1769, 2007

Ingerski LM, Anderson BJ, Dolan LM, Hood KK: Blood glucose monitoring and glycemic control in adolescence: contribution of diabetes-specific responsibility and family conflict. *J Adolesc Health* 47:191–197, 2010

Jones JM, Bennett S, Olmsted MP, Lawson ML, Rodin G: Disordered eating attitudes and behaviours in teenaged girls: a school-based study. *CMAJ* 165:547–552, 2001

Jones JM, Lawson ML, Daneman D, Olmsted MP, Rodin G: Eating disorders in adolescent females with and without type 1 diabetes: cross sectional study. *BMJ* 320:1563–1566, 2000

Kipps S, Bahu T, Ong K, Acklandt F, Brown R, Fox C, Griffin N, Knight A, Mann N, Simpson H, Edge J, Dunger D: Current methods of transfer of young people with type 1 diabetes to adult services. *Diabet Med* 19:649–654, 2002

Kitabchi AE, Umpierrez GE, Miles JM, Fisher JN: Hyperglycemia crises in adult patients with diabetes. *Diabetes Care* 32:1335–1343, 2009

Kovacs M, Goldston D, Obrosky DS, Bonar LK: Psychiatric disorders in youths with IDDM: rates and risk factors. *Diabetes Care* 20:36–44, 1997

Kumar VS, Wentzell KJ, Mikkelsen T, Pentland A, Laffel LM: The DAILY (Daily Automated Intensive Log for Youth) trial: a wireless, portable system to improve adherence and glycemic control in youth with diabetes. *Diabetes Technol Ther* 6:445–453, 2004

Lara A: Animal lover's guide to kids: why tots are like puppies and teens are like cats. *Working Mother* November:88, 1996

Lehmkuhl H, Merlo L, Devine K, Gaines J, Storch E, Silverstien J, Gefken G: Perceptions of type 1 diabetes among affected youth and their peers. *J Clin Psychol Med Settings* 16:209–215, 2009

Lewinsohn PM, Rohde P, Seeley JR, Klein DN, Gotlib IH: Natural course of adolescent major depressive disorder in a community sample: predictors of recurrence in young adults. *Am J Psychiatry* 157:1584–1591, 2000

Lilenfeld SO: Scientifically unsupported and supported interventions for childhood psychopathology: a summary. *Pediatrics* 115:761–764, 2005

LoCasale-Crouch J, Johnson B: Transition from pediatric to adult medical care. *Adv Chronic Kidney Dis* 12:412–417, 2005

Lotstein DS, Ghandour R, Cash A, McGuire E, Strickland B, Newacheck P: Planning for health care transitions: results from the 2005-2006 National Survey of Children with Special Health Care Needs. *Pediatrics* 123:e145–e152, 2009

Lotstein DS, McPherson M, Strickland B, Newacheck PW: Transition planning for youth with special health care needs: results from the National Survey of Children with Special Health Care Needs. *Pediatrics* 115:1562–1568, 2005

Malik JA, Koot HM: Assessing diabetes support in adolescents: factor structure of the modified diabetes social support questionnaire. *Diabet Med* 29:e232–e240, 2012

March J, Silva S, Petrycki S, Curry J, Wells K, Fairbank J, Burns B, Domino M, McNulty S, Vitiello B, Severe J; Treatment for Adolescents With Depression Study (TADS) Team: Fluoxetine, cognitive-behavioral therapy, and their combination for adolescents with depression: Treatment for Adolescents With Depression Study (TADS) randomized controlled trial. *JAMA* 292:807–820, 2004

Markowitz JT, Lowe MR, Laffel LMB: Self-reported history of overweight and its relationship to disordered eating in adolescent girls with type 1 diabetes. *Diabet Med* 26:1165–1171, 2009

McDonagh JE, Southwood TR, Shaw KL: The impact of a coordinated transitional care programme on adolescents with juvenile idiopathic arthritis. *Rheumatology* 46:161–168, 2007

Merton RK: *Social Theory and Social Structure.* New York, Free Press, 1968

Miller KM, Beck RW, Bergenstal RM, Goland RS, Haller MJ, McGill JB, Rodriguez H, Simmons JH, Hirsch IB: Evidence of a strong association between frequency of self-monitoring of blood glucose and hemoglobin A1c levels in T1D exchange clinic registry participants. *Diabetes Care* 36:2009–2014, 2013

Mulvaney SA, Anders S, Smith AK, Pittel EJ, Johnson KB: A pilot test of a tailored mobile and web-based diabetes messaging system for adolescents. *J Telemed Telecare* 18:115–118, 2012

Nakhla M, Daneman D, Frank M, Guttman A: Translating transition: a critical review of the diabetes literature. *Diabetes Technol Ther* 11:211–217, 2009

Neu A, Losch-Binder M, Ehehalt S, Schweizer R, Hub R, Serra E: Follow-up of adolescents with diabetes after transition from pediatric to adult care: results of a 10-year prospective study. *Exp Clin Endocrinol Diabetes* 118:353–355, 2010

Nickerson RS: Confirmation bias: a ubiquitous phenomenon in many guises. *Rev Gen Psychol* 2:175–220, 1998

Office of Disease Prevention and Health Promotion, U.S. Department of Health and Human Services: *Healthy People 2010*. www.healthypeople.gov

Olinder AL, Kernell A, Smide B: Missed bolus doses: devastating for metabolic control in CSII-treated adolescents with type 1 diabetes. *Pediatric Diabetes* 10:142–148, 2009

Olmsted MP, Colton PA, Daneman D, Rydall AC, Rodin GM: Prediction of the onset of disturbed eating behavior in adolescent girls with type 1 diabetes. *Diabetes Care* 31:1978–1982, 2008

Osterberg L, Blaschke T: Adherence to medication. *N Engl J Med* 353:487–497, 2005

Peters A, Laffel L; American Diabetes Association Transitions Working Group: Diabetes care for emerging adults: recommendations for transition from pediatric to adult diabetes care systems: a position statement of the American Diabetes Association. *Diabetes Care* 34:2477–2485, 2011

Petitti D, Klingensmith G, Bell R, Andrews J, Dabelea D, Imperatore G, Marcovina S, Pihoker C, Standiford D, Waitzfelder B, Mayer-Davis E, for the SEARCH for Diabetes in Youth Study Group: Glycemic control in youth with diabetes: the SEARCH for Diabetes in Youth Study. *J Pediatr* 155:668–672, 2009

Peveler RC, Bryden KS, Neil HA, Fairburn CG, Mayou RA, Dunger DB, Turner HM: The relationship of disordered eating habits and attitudes to clinical outcomes in young adult females with type 1 diabetes. *Diabetes Care* 28:84–88, 2005

Phillip M, Battleino T, Rodriguez H, Dane T, Kaufman F: Use of insulin pump therapy in the pediatric age-group. *Diabetes Care* 30:1653–1662, 2007

Raile K, Noelle V, Landgraf R, Schwarz HP: Weight in adolescents with type 1 diabetes mellitus during continuous subcutaneous insulin infusion (CSII) therapy. *J Pediatr Endocrinol Metab* 15:607–612, 2002

Regber SS, Berg K, Kelly KB: Missed opportunities: adolescents with a chronic condition (insulin-dependent diabetes mellitus) describe their cigarette-smoking trajectories and consider health risks. *Acta Paediatr* 96:1770–1776, 2007

Reiss J, Gibson R, Walker L: Health care transition: youth, family, and provider perspectives. *Pediatrics* 115:112–120, 2005

Reynolds K, Liese AD, Anderson AM, Dabelea D, et al.: Prevalence of tobacco use and association between cardiometabolic risk factors and cigarette smoking in youth with type 1 or type 2 diabetes mellitus. *J Pediatr* 158:594–601, 2011

Roberts GC, Block JH, Block J: Continuity and change in parents' child-rearing practices. *Child Dev* 55:586–597, 1984

Robin A, Foster SL: *Negotiating Parent-Adolescent Conflict*. New York, Guilford Press, 1989

Ross L: The intuitive psychologist and his shortcomings: distortions in the attribution process. In Berkowitz L. *Advances in Experimental Social Psychology*. New York, Academic Press, 1977, p. 173–220

Royal College of Pediatrics and Child Health: *Bridging the Gaps: Health Care for Adolescents*. London, Royal College of Pediatrics and Child Health, 2003

Rydall AC, Rodin GM, Olmsted MP, Devenyi RG, Daneman D: Disordered eating behavior and microvascular complications in young women with insulin-dependent diabetes mellitus. *N Engl J Med* 336:1849–1854, 1997

Scal P, Evans T, Blozis S, Okinow N, Blum R: Trends in transition from pediatric to adult health care services for young adults with chronic conditions. *J Adolesc Health* 24:259–264, 1999

Society for Adolescent Medicine: Transition to adult health care for adolescent and young adults with chronic conditions. *J Adolesc Health* 33:309–311, 2003

Sparud-Lundin C, Ohrn I, Danielson E, Forsander G: Glycemic control and diabetes care utilization in young adults with type 1 diabetes. *Diabet Med* 25:968–973, 2008

Street RL, Makoul G, Arora NK, Epstein RM: How does communication heal? Pathways linking clinician-patient communication to health outcomes. *Patient Educ Couns* 74:295–301, 2009

Telfair J, Myers J, Drezner S: Transfer as a component of the transition of adolescent with sickle cell disease to adult care: adolescents, adult and parent perspective. *J Adolesc Health* 15:558–565, 1994

VanWalleghem N, Macdonald C, Dean H: Evaluation of a systems navigator model for transition from pediatric to adult care for young adults with type 1 diabetes. *Diabetes Care* 31:1529–1530, 2008

VanWalleghem N, MacDonald CA, Dean HJ: Building connections for young adults with type 1 diabetes mellitus in Manitoba: feasibility and acceptability of a transition initiative. *Chronic Dis Can* 27:130–134, 2006

Weibe D, Berg C, Korgel C, et al.: Children's appraisal of maternal involvement in coping with diabetes: enhancing our understanding of adherence, glycemic control, and quality of life across adolescence. *J Pediatr Psychol* 30:167–178, 2005

Weissberg-Benchell J, Nansel T, Holmbeck G, Chen R, Anderson B, Wysocki T, Laffel L: Generic versus diabetes-specific quality of life and parent-child behaviors among youth with type 1 diabetes. *J Pediatr Psychol* 34:977–988, 2009

Westwood A, Henley L, Wilcox P: Transition from paediatric to adult care for persons with cystic fibrosis: patient and parent perspective. *J Paediatr Child Health* 35:442–445, 1999

Williams LB, Laffel L, Hood K: Diabetes-specific family conflict and psychological distress in paediatric type 1 diabetes. *Diabet Med* 26:908–914, 2009

Wills CJ, Swift PGF, Davies MJ, Mackie ADR, Mansell P: Retrospective review of care and outcome in young adults with type 1 diabetes. *BMJ* 327:260–261, 2003

Wojciechowski E, Hurtig Al, Dorn L: A natural history study of adolescent and young adults with sickle cell disease as they transfer to adult care: a need for case management services. *J Pediatr Nurs* 17:18–22, 2002

Wysocki T: Associations among teen-parent relationships, metabolic control, and adjustment to diabetes in adolescents. *J Pediatr Psychol* 18:441–452, 1992

Wysocki T, Greco P: Social support and diabetes management in childhood and adolescence: influence of parents and friends. *Curr Diab Rep* 6: 117–122, 2006

Wysocki T, Harris MA, Buckloh LM, Mertlich D, Lochrie AS, Mauras N, White NH: Randomized trial of behavioral family systems therapy for diabetes: maintenance of effects on adolescents' diabetes outcomes. *Diabetes Care* 30:555–560, 2007

Wysocki T, Harris MA, Greco P, Bubb J, Elder CL, Harvey LM, McDonell K, Taylor A, White NH: Randomized controlled trial of behavior therapy for families of adolescents with insulin-dependent diabetes mellitus. *J Pediatr Psychol* 25:23–33, 2000

Wysocki T, Harris M, Greco P, Harvey L, McDonell K, Danda C, Bubb J, White N: Social validity of support group and behavior therapy interventions for families of adolescents with insulin-dependent diabetes mellitus. *J Pediatr Psychol* 22:635–649, 1997

Wysocki T, Harris MA, Greco P, Mertlich D, Buckloh LM: *Behavioral Family Systems Therapy for Adolescents with Diabetes: Treatment and Implementation Manual.* Unpublished treatment manual, 2001

Wysocki T, Miller KM, Greco P, Harris MA, Harvey LM, Elder-Danda CL, Taylor A, McDonell K, White NH: Behavior therapy for families of adolescents with diabetes: effects on directly observed family interactions. *Behavior Therapy* 30:496–515, 1999

Wysocki T, Nansel T, Holmbeck G, et al.: Collaborative involvement of primary and secondary caregivers: associations with youth's diabetes outcomes. *J Pediatr Psychol* 34:869–881, 2009

Yu H, Wier LM, Elizhauser A: *Hospital Stays for Children, 2006.* HUCP Statistical Brief #118. Rockville, MD, Agency for Healthcare Research and Quality, 2011

Index

JUN 2 5 2015

Date Due

BRODART, CO.   Cat. No. 23-233   Printed in U.S.A.